Prevention of Disease in the Elderly

MEDICINE IN OLD AGE

Editorial Advisory Board

Bernard Isaacs MD, FRCP
Charles Hayward Professor of Geriatric Medicine,
University of Birmingham

J.C. Brocklehurst MD, MSc, FRCP
Professor of Geriatric Medicine,
University of Manchester

Robert W. Stout MD, FRCP
Professor of Geriatric Medicine, The Queen's
University of Belfast

Brice Pitt MD, MRCPsych, DPM
Consultant Psychiatrist,
The London Hospital

T. Franklin Williams MD
Director, National Institute of Aging, Bethesda,
Maryland

Marc E. Weksler BA MD
Wright Professor of Medicine,
Cornell University Medical College, New York

Volumes already published

Hearing and balance in the elderly
R. Hinchcliffe, *Editor*

Bone and joint disease in the elderly
V. Wright, *Editor*

Peripheral vascular disease in the elderly
S.T. McCarthy, *Editor*

Clinical pharmacology and drug treatment in the elderly
K. O'Malley, *Editor*

Clinical biochemistry in the elderly
H.M. Hodkinson, *Editor*

Immunology and infection in the elderly
R.A. Fox, *Editor*

Gastrointestinal tract disorders in the elderly
J. Hellemans and G. Vantrappen, *Editors*

Arterial disease in the elderly
R.W. Stout, *Editor*

Blood disorders in the elderly
M.J. Denham and I. Chanarin, *Editors*

Volumes in preparation

Cardiology in the elderly
R.J. Luchi, *Editor*

Medical ethics and the elderly
R.J. Elford, *Editor*

Affective disorders in the elderly
E. Murphy, *Editor*

Dementia
B. Pit, *Editor*

Psychological assessment of the elderly
J.P. Wattis and I. Hindmarch

Prevention of Disease in the Elderly

Edited by

J.A. Muir Gray
MD MRCGP MRCP FFCM
Community Physician,
Oxfordshire Health Authority, Oxford, UK

CHURCHILL LIVINGSTONE
EDINBURGH LONDON MELBOURNE AND NEW YORK 1985

CHURCHILL LIVINGSTONE
Medical Division of Longman Group Limited

Distributed in the United States of America by
Churchill Livingstone Inc., 1560 Broadway, New York,
N.Y. 10036, and by associated companies, branches
and representatives throughout the world.

© Longman Group Limited 1985

All rights reserved. No part of this publication
may be reproduced, stored in a retrieval system,
or transmitted in any form or by any means,
electronic, mechanical, photocopying, recording
or otherwise, without the prior permission of the
publishers (Churchill Livingstone, Robert Stevenson
House, 1-3 Baxter's Place, Leith Walk,
Edinburgh EH1 3AF).

First published 1985

ISBN 0 443 02962 8
ISSN 0264-5602

British Library Cataloguing in Publication Data
Prevention of disease in the elderly. — (Medicine
  in old age, ISSN 0264–5602)
  1. Aged — Diseases 2. Medicine, Preventive
  I. Gray, Muir II. Series
  613'.0438   RC952.5

Library of Congress Cataloging in Publication Data
Prevention of disease in the elderly.
  (Medicine in old age, ISSN 0264–5602)
  Includes index.
  1. Aged — Diseases — Prevention. 2. Medicine,
Preventive. I. Gray, J.A. Muir (John Armstrong Muir)
II. Series. [DNLM: 1. Geriatrics. 2. Primary
Prevention — in old age. WT 100 P944]
  RA564.8.P74   1985   618.97   85–6635

Printed and Bound in Gt. Britain at The Bath Press,
Avon

To Tink, Tat and Jackie with love

Acknowledgement

I should like to thank Mrs Rosemary Lees, my secretary, who has helped me so much in the preparation of this book.

Introduction

To a great extent the medicine of today and tomorrow is the medicine of old age. In every hospital in the Western World old patients predominate. In the past it was too readily assumed that either the medicine of old age was confined to degenerative disease and was uninfluenced by diagnosis and treatment; or that it was identical to the medicine of young and middle age and required no special study. Neither view is correct. It is now becoming clear that the diseases which strike old people, the symptoms and the signs which are induced, and the response to treatment are distinctive. Years of growth, maturation and decline alter the response of the host to disease and to its management in ways which require special study. As this fact has been grasped medical science and research-minded clinicians have embarked on the study of the diseases of late life and have documented their characteristic features. Progress has been slow, partly because of an initial lack of sense of urgency, and difficulty in attracting research workers and funds; partly because of the complexities of defining normal values in old age and of attributing deviations from the normal to any one cause. Methodological and statistical problems have compounded the difficulties. But over the years there has been a very real and impressive growth of knowledge of the medicine of late life.

Some years ago the idea was conceived of collecting this new knowledge, system by system, in a series of volumes to be entitled 'Medicine in Old Age'. These books were addressed to physicians in all Western countries and in all medical disciplines who dealt with elderly patients. The contributors included physiologists, pathologists, epidemiologists and community physicians, as well as general internal physicians, geriatricians, psychiatrists and specialists in the various systems of the body. The response accorded to the first few volumes in the series was most encouraging, and the publishers are continuing and expanding the series.

This enterprise is supervised by an Editorial Board composed of practising clinicians and academics on both sides of the Atlantic. The Board selects the topics and appoints the guest editors for each volume and have been fortunate in their choice as editors of leaders in each field. These have been able in turn to attract contributions of high merit from many countries, thus putting into the hands of the reader a series of highly authoritative volumes. These bring together a wealth of knowledge and the best of modern practice in the care of elderly patients, retaining the critical spirit in the evaluation of the data which is characteristic of medicine in all age groups. The volumes are intended to stand mid-way between the immediacy of the scientific journal and the urbanity of the standard text book, combining freshness with authority. It is hoped that the profession will find them of value.

Bernard Isaacs

Preface

In the last decade it has become clearer and clearer that many of the changes that are more common in old age are not the inevitable consequences of biological ageing but result from having lived a long life exposed to certain risk factors. The increasing incidence of cancer with age, for example, is not due to the effects of normal ageing but to the simple fact that old people have been exposed to carcinogens for longer than young people. There is accumulating evidence that many of the disorders that occur in old age are preventable and my intention in this book has been to bring together some of this evidence and to summarise and analyse some of the ways in which this knowledge can be applied. I have tried to concentrate on measures that can be taken after one has reached the age of seventy but foundations of good health in old age are, of course, laid not only in one's genes but also in childhood and early adult life.

Hitherto the term 'prevention' has had connotations of youth but the scope for prevention in old age is so great that I believe that we will see increasing emphasis on prevention in old age in the next decade. There is concern about the effects of such a policy, notably the belief that it will increase the numbers of very severely disabled older people, but my own view is that we are already seeing a dramatic rise in the numbers of such people, an increase resulting from social and economic changes in times past and not from preventive policies aimed at middle-aged and older people. Accepting that the numbers of older people are increasing our objective must therefore be to minimise the incidence and prevalence of disability and handicap and this book demonstrates how reductions can be achieved. The objective of prevention in old age is not to prolong life but to heelp people live well, to help people, in Richard Doll's words when asked his ambition, to 'die young as late as possible'.

Oxford   MUIR GRAY
1985

Contributors

G. Almind
General Practitioners, Holback, Denmark

Sandra L. Baker MB ChB(Hons) MRCP
Consultant Geriatrician, Dudley Road Hospital, Birmingham, UK

E. Joan Bassey BSc PhD
Lecturer, University of Nottingham Medical School, Nottingham, UK

Charles B. Freer MB ChB MClSc MRCGP
Senior Lecturer, Primary Medical Care, University of Southampton, UK

Jeffrey Garland BA DipAppPsych DPhil
Principal Clinical Psychologist, Care of the Elderly, Oxford District Health Authority, Oxford, UK

J.A. Muir Gray MD MRCGP MRCP (Glas) FFCM
Community Physician, Oxfordshire Health Authority, Radcliffe Infirmary, Oxford, UK

James D.E. Knox MD FRCGP FRCP(Ed)
Head of Department of General Practice, University of Dundee, UK

R. Lindsay PhD MRCP
Chief Executive Officer, Helen Hayes Hospital, New York, USA

Hamish N. Munro MD DSc
Former Director, USDA Human Nutrition Research Center for Aging, and Professor of Medicine, Tufts University, Boston, USA; Professor of Physiological Chemistry, Massachussetts Institute of Technology, Cambridge, USA

Elaine Murphy MB ChB MD MRCPsych
Professor of Psychogeriatrics, Guy's Hospital Medical School, London, UK

Alan Pearson MSc RGN ONC RNT DipNEd DipAdvNStud
Senior Nurse, Clinical Practice, Community Unit, Oxfordshire Health Authority, Oxford, UK

Peter Sandercock MA (Oxon) BM BCh MRCP
Clinical Lecturer in Neurology, Radcliffe Infirmary, Oxford, UK

Charles Warlow MD FRCP
Clinical Reader in Neurology, University of Oxford, UK

G. Warshaw MD
Assistant Professor of Family Medicine, Duke University, Nortt Caroline, USA

Archie Young BSc MD MRCP
Clinical Lecturer/Honorary Consultant Physician, University of Oxford, UK

Contents

1	The scope for prevention *J.A. Muir Gray*	1
2	Prevention of dependency *Jeffrey Garland*	18
3	The prevention of family breakdown *J.A. Muir Gray*	38
4	Screening and case finding *C. Freer, G. Almind, G. Warshaw and J.A. Muir Gray*	51
5	Prevention of iatrogenic disease *J.D.E. Knox*	64
6	The risks of inactivity *J.A. Muir Gray, E.J. Bassey and A. Young*	78
7	Prevention of osteoporosis *Robert Lindsay*	95
8	The preventability of falls *Sandra L. Baker*	114
9	The prevention of stroke in the elderly *Peter Sandercock and Charles Warlow*	130
10	Prevention of depression and suicide *Elaine Murphy*	156
11	Nutritional aspects of ageing: present status and implications *Hamish N. Munro*	178
12	Prevention of pressure sores *Alan Pearson*	194
13	Education for health in old age *J.A. Muir Gray*	214
	Index	227

1   *J. A. Muir Gray*

The scope for prevention

OBJECTIVES OF PREVENTION IN OLD AGE

The achievements of preventive medicine have been widely publicised in recent years, and the decline in both adult and child mortality rates has been attributed to preventive measures. The focus of preventive interest still remains principally on mortality, on reducing the mortality from cancer and heart disease, but attention is turning to the prevention of disability, in addition to the prevention of premature death. This trend is of particular relevance for older people, for there is little professional or public interest in prolonging the life in old age: most people are interest in quality of life rather than quantity. Thus the objective of prevention in old age is not to reduce mortality rates, and other objectives have therefore to be identified.

The Surgeon General of the United States suggested such a goal in his report on health promotion and disease preventing, *Healthy People* (U.S. Department of Health Education & Welfare, 1979): 'To improve the health and quality of life for older adults and, by 1990, to reduce the average annual number of days of restricted activity due to acute and chronic conditions by 20 per cent to fewer than 30 days per year for people aged 65 and older.' This objective, however, covers only one aspect of health in old age, and other objectives can also be identified as a basis for service planning and evaluation, for example:
1. To prevent a decline in the quality of life
2. To prevent family breakdown
3. To keep elderly people in their homes as long as possible, if that is what they wish.

These are also vaguely worded statements and it is essential that they be quantified, but they are appropriate objectives on which to plan a preventive strategy.

THE SCOPE FOR PREVENTION

The scope for prevention has not been quantified precisely. Evidence has to be drawn from a number of sources.

Evidence from mortality data

Although the objective of prevention in old age is not to prolong life mortality, data suggest that there is considerable scope for prevention in old age, for two reasons.
1. Mortality rates of old people differ from one country to another (Table 1.1).
2. There has been a decline in the mortality rates in old age in all developed countries (Fig. 1.1).

The difference in mortality rates of men and women also suggests that there is scope for prevention, for there is now evidence that the difference between the sexes is not due solely to genetic factors. Other factors, notably the different prevalence of cigarette smoking, are also of importance. As with the decline in mortality in childhood and early adult life, the decline in mortality in old age has been too rapid to be due to genetic evolution and must be due to either more effective treatment of disease or more effective prevention, or to both, and the consensus is that prevention of disease has been more important than treatment in reducing mortality (McKeown, 1979).

Mortality and morbidity

The fact that death can be postponed does not of course prove that disability can be prevented or that any of the other objectives listed in the first section can be attained, because the relationship between mortality and morbidity is not clear.

Fries has argued that the 'rectangularisation of the survival curve' illustrated in Figure 1.2 is accompanied by a 'compression of morbidity', namely a decline in the period of time in which a person is severely disabled in old age.

Table 1.1 Changes in mortality among the elderly in the United States, 1940–78 (US Department of Health and Human Service: Office of Health Research Statistics and Technology. Analytical Studies Series 3, No. 22)

	Death rates per 1000 in 1977			
	70–74 years		75–79 years	
	Men	Women	Men	Women
Japan	46.2	27.3	77.0	51.1
Sweden	47.1	25.2	77.9	47.8
Canada	50.6	26.4	75.5	42.4
France	51.3	24.1	84.4	45.7
Netherlands	52.4	25.5	78.1	46.8
United States	53.2	27.7	81.5	47.4
Australia	55.7	28.7	85.8	50.7
West Germany	61.8	32.5	94.4	58.8
England	62.3	32.1	96.1	54.9

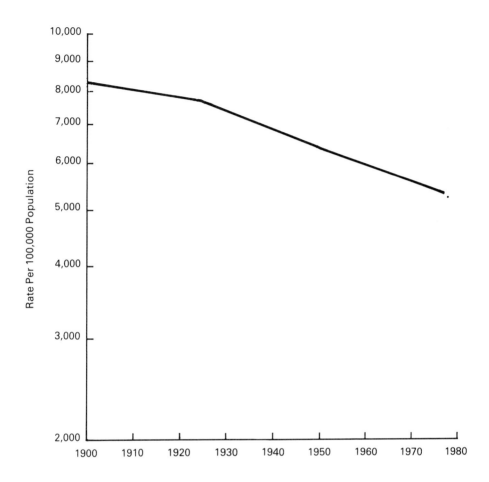

Note: 1977 data are provisional; data for all other years are final.
Selected years are 1900, 1925, 1950, 1977.

Fig. 1.1 Death rates for ages 65 years and over: United States, selected years 1900–77 (National Center for Health Statistics, Division of Vital Statistics)

However, the rectangularisation of the survival curve for a whole population is not necessarily reflected in the rectangularisation of the decline curve for individuals within that population. Others are more pessimistic and maintain that the effect of the increase in life expectancy is to prolong the period of terminal disability and dependency (Schneider & Brody, 1983).

Mortality data are inadequate for the analysis of this issue and other approaches have to be used.

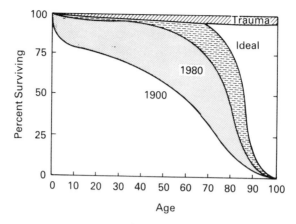

Fig. 1.2 American survival curves in 1900, 1980 and in ideal circumstances (Fries, 1980)

Gerontological evidence

Basic research into the process of ageing is still at an early stage but it is now clear that the changes that occur with age are not due to the ageing process alone. Three other interrelated processes are also responsible:
1. Loss of fitness
2. Social changes, such as the drop in income on retirement
3. Pathological processes.

These three processes, unlike the ageing process, are modifiable and thus the idea that all the problems of old age are inevitable has been replaced by the acceptance of the idea that a proportion are preventable.

In general, the more that is known about the problems of old age the less are they seen to be due to the ageing process, and the 80-year-old person who is affected by the ageing process alone will be active and lively and have an enjoyable life.

Evidence from population surveys

The medical view of old age has for a long time been heavily influenced by the fact that doctors see sick people. They thus associate old age with sickness. However, studies of whole populations of old people revealed a different perspective, as Seebohm Rowntree's committee on the *Problems of Ageing* (Rowntree, 1947) stated in 1947 when commenting on Sheldon's classic study of old people in Wolverhampton (Sheldon, 1948) that his survey 'although a medical survey will in fact turn out to be a survey of health, for the toughness and resilience of many of these old people is remarkable'.

This type of cross-sectional study has an important defect because the fact that differences are demonstrated between different age groups may lead to the conclusion that the cause of these differences is solely the ageing process.

On the basis of a number of studies the relationship between a number of variables and age has been displayed on diagrames such as Figure 1.3.

The assumption that may be made from such data is that the decline in function is due to the ageing process alone. For some organs this may be the case; for others it is not, as more sophisticated studies can demonstrate, for example the definition of subgroups within the total population allows the influence of other factors to be demonstrated (Fig. 1.4).

Similarly cross-sectional studies of intelligence give the impression that there is a marked decline in intelligence with age, whereas the difference between 30-year-olds and 80-year-olds is not due simply to the ageing process. Other factors, notably the amount of formal education experienced by the two groups, are also relevant. A cross-sectional study, therefore, gives a

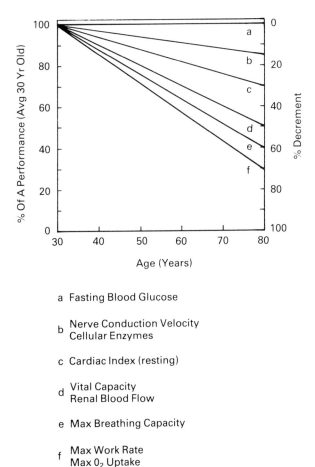

a Fasting Blood Glucose

b Nerve Conduction Velocity
  Cellular Enzymes

c Cardiac Index (resting)

d Vital Capacity
  Renal Blood Flow

e Max Breathing Capacity

f Max Work Rate
  Max O₂ Uptake

Fig.1.3 Decrements in physiological function in normal men aged 30 to 80 years (expressed as a percentage of average values for 30-year-olds) (American Association for Clinical Chemistry, 1979)

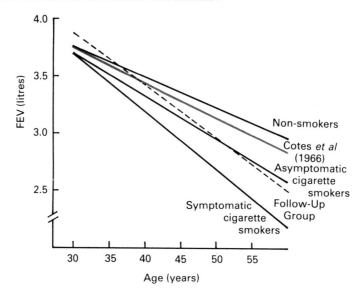

Fig.1.4 Changes in forced expiratory volume with age (Fletcher et al, 1976)

misleading impression of the effects of the ageing process. If studies are designed to follow one group of people throughout their life — longitudinal studies — then a different picture is obtained (Fig. 1.5).

Evidence from longitudinal studies

Surveys of the whole population — cross-sectional studies — reveal that many old people are healthy and well and provide more evidence that there is scope for prevention than clinical data, but longitudinal studies in which the same group of people is followed as its members grow old are even more useful than cross-sectional studies.

They are, however, difficult and expensive to carry out, as Shephard has graphically described. (Shephard, 1978):

> The longitudinal approach also has its problems. The interest of subjects must be secured and maintained over a long period, and this predisposes to recruitment of a health-conscious minority of the total population. Some of the sample will develop inter-current disease, and must then be eliminated. Ideally, observers and techniques should remain constant throughout the study. The apparent magnitude of something as simple as a skinfold thickness can change by up to 25 per cent if it is measured by a different technician or even a different design of fat caliper. If the constancy of methodology is assured, there remains the hazard that laboratory procedures considered acceptable at the outset of an investigation will have become seriously dated before all of the required information has been collected. Finally, the enthusiasm of the principal investigator must be preserved and the impatience of the granting agency must be withstood over the long period while figures are accumulating.

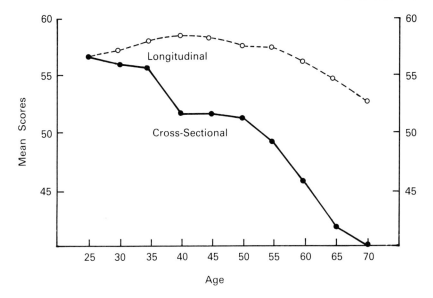

Fig. 1.5 Results of a cross-sectional study of intelligence measured in groups of people of different ages compared with the decline in intelligence that would be observed if the same group were followed and tested every five years for forty-five years (Schaie & Strother, 1968)

The costs are high, but the benefits are great. Firstly, a longitudinal study of a cohort which demonstrates a different rate of decline with age than is observed in a cross-sectional sample suggests that the difference between the different age groups cannot be assumed to be due simply to the ageing process. If it were, the rate of decline of a single cohort would be the same as the decline observed in the whole population at a cross-sectional study. If it is not, then factors which specifically affect each cohort have to be taken into consideration (Fig. 1.6).

In this example, the difference in heights between 30-year-olds and 60-year-olds is not simply due to the fact that the latter have been affected by the ageing process for thirty years more than the former: it is due to the fact that the cohort of 60-year-olds was, on average, smaller in childhood than the cohort of 30-year-olds, for social and economic, and not biological, reasons.

In spite of the difficulties, a number of longitudinal studies have been set up, notably the studies in Göteborg, in Sweden, Glostrup, in Denmark, and the Duke University Study in North Carolina, USA, and these studies are starting to produce very useful results.

The problems of single-cohort studies

The simplest type of longitudinal study is that in which a single cohort of people born in the same year is followed. This type of study usefully comple-

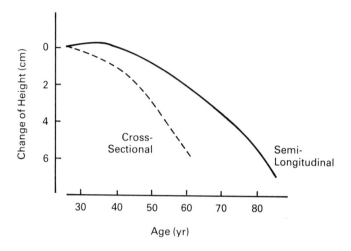

Fig. 1.6 Differences in the rate of change of standing height with age as seen in semi-longitudinal and cross-sectional data. Observation of Miall et al (1967) on men living in the Rhondda Fach

ments the cross-sectional study, but it is difficult to draw general conclusions about the effects of ageing from the study of a single cohort.

For example, any study of physical activity in old age has to take into account not only the effects of ageing and the influence on the cohort at an early stage in its life. It also has to take into account the changing environment in which that cohort has lived; in the case of exercise a social and physical environment in which physical activity has declined at all ages and the artefacts produced by both cross-sectional and single cohort longitudinal studies are clearly illustrated in Figure 1.7. Such secular trends are common and some of them are very important, for example the increasing consumption of cigarettes and the decrease in concentration of particulate pollution in the atmosphere.

There are thus three types of factor which influence the rate of decline: factors affecting all cohorts, factors specific to one cohort, and secular changes in the different social or physical environment which have different effects on different cohorts. It is therefore essential to study more than one cohort if the relationship between ageing, factors affecting one particular cohort, and general environmental factors is to be elucidated. The Göteborg study now includes more than one cohort; 1148 seventy-year-olds were recruited in 1971, 1281 seventy-year-olds were recruited in 1977, and a third cohort was recruited in 1982. It is this type of approach which is required if the natural history of old age is to be understood (Svanborg et al, 1982; Busse & Maddox, 1982). However, this method is obviously very expensive, and statistical techniques have been developed which allow studies of a number of cohorts to be done more cheaply. The two types of method that are most commonly employed are retrospective cohort analysis and cross-sequential analysis.

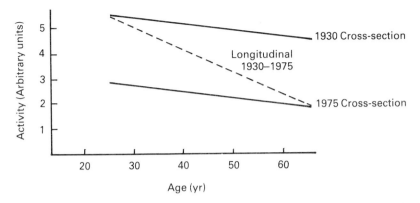

Fig.1.7 The influence of a secular trend to reduced habitual activity. In a longitudinal study, the usual decline of physical activity with age is exaggerated (Shephard, 1978)

Retrospective cohort analysis

Mortality data are usually presented by age at death and year of death. If, however, they are presented by year of birth by cohort, a different picture may emerge. This technique has been used to demonstrate that the higher mortality rates from tuberculosis in old age do not reflect an increased incidence with age, and that even in the oldest age groups the mortality rate is actually declining (Fig. 1.8).

Cross-sequential analysis

Techniques have been developed which allow the changes that will occur in a whole series of cohorts to be predicted. The 'longitudinal' curve depicting the decline in intelligence in Figure 1.2 is in fact based on the short-term follow-ups of a large number of cohorts. The rate of decline between the two assessments is calculated for each cohort, and from these data a curve such as that which could be obtained by following a small number of cohorts for a large number of years is obtained. This has been called the cross-sequential technique and has been developed to allow the three types of factors that determine the rate of decline in old age to be distinguished from another with less cost and, it must be emphasised, less accuracy than the formal techniques used in the Göteborg study. These three types of factor are:
1. Ageing factors, common to all cohorts.
2. Factors specific to one cohort.
3. Extrinsic factors common to all cohorts, such as the decline in activity levels in developed societies.

The scope for prevention in old age

The scope for prevention of many of the problems of old age is considerable,

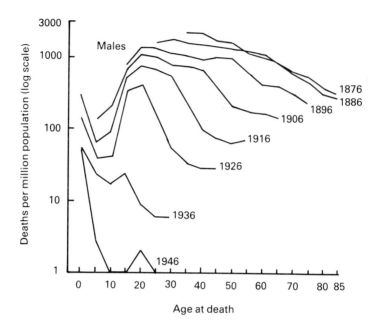
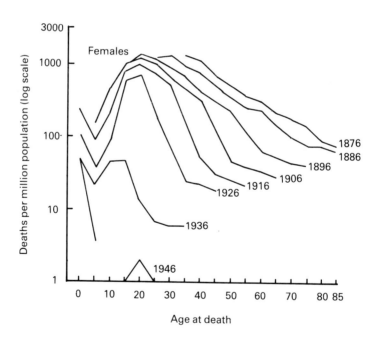

Fig. 1.8 Pulmonary tuberculosis: annual death rates by age in selected cohorts, 1920–75, England and Wales (Adelstein, 1977)

but for full effectiveness preventive measures have to start in childhood and continue throughout adult life. Old age is not a separate stage in life; it is a part of a continuum, and health in old age is part of the continuum of health. One other point of great importance is that there also appears to be scope for prevention even when a person has reached old age. Most of the evidence on the scope for prevention in old age has come from the study of the effects of exercise in old age (Shephard, 1978), but the message that is emerging from a number of different fields of study is that it is never too late for prevention.

THE TIMING OF PREVENTION

One of the characteristics of the preventive approach is the importance of the natural history of a disease, and three stages in the development of a disease can usually be identified:
1. The period in which the individual does not have the disease; in some diseases risk factors can be identified at this stage.
2. The asymptomatic stage.
3. The symptomatic stage.

These three stages provide the basis for the classification of preventive interventions into three main types. These are usually known as primary, secondary and tertiary prevention.

Primary prevention

The WHO glossary of health terms defines primary prevention as being 'all measures designed to reduce the incidence of disease in a population by reducing the risk of onset'. This term is used universally.

Secondary prevention

The WHO definition for secondary prevention is that it consists of 'all measures designed to reduce the prevalence of a disease in a population by shortening its course and duration'. The term, however, is not widely used now. It has been superseded by two other terms: screening and case-finding. Both these terms also have WHO definitions. Screening is the identification of an 'unrecognised disease or defect' in 'apparently well persons'. Case-finding aims to detect established disease which has not previously been reported to the health services (Wilson & Jungner, 1968).

Both these approaches therefore detect hidden needs, but in screening the objective is to detect asymptomatic disease or the asymptomatic precursor of disease, whereas in case-finding the objective is to detect problems of which the elderly person is aware but which have previously been unreported or undetected by health-care professionals.

Tertiary prevention

This is simply effective clinical intervention, and one of the most important developments in clinical work in the last ten years has been the growing appreciation of the fact that the acute and chronic diseases in old age can be effectively treated. A number of characteristics of disease in old age have been identified which are of particular relevance to clinical practice, for example the fact that presentation is frequently atypical and the fact that deterioration may occur more quickly than in younger people. However, certain aspects of disease in old age are of relevance for prevention, notably:
1. The effects of immobilisation are much more severe in old age.
2. Hospitalisation more frequently has an adverse effect in old age.
3. Recovery is slower in old age and complete recovery may never be attained.

For these reasons the prevention of disease is of particular importance in old age, even though the clinical management of disease is much more effective than it was ten or twenty years ago.

THE MEANS OF PREVENTION

Diseases are prevented by a variety of different approaches, but the various means of prevention can be grouped into four inter-related processes (Fig. 1.9).

Health education

In the past the assumption was that people were ignorant about disease, and health education was simply seen as the provision of health information to the ignorant. This is now known to be an inaccurate assumption and an ineffective approach. Old people are not ignorant about health. They know a lot about health; they have beliefs and attitudes which they find satisfactory. This is not to argue that they are complacent. Most elderly people want the opportunity to learn more about their health but they do not simply want to be the passive recipients of information about disease. Any health education that is to be effective must
1. be based on the beliefs of elderly people
2. involve them as active participants
3. take into account the relevant social and political factors that influence health in old age.

Health education should not only consist of advice on lifestyle; it should relate to the other aspects of prevention by
1. giving advice on the appropriate use of personal preventive services
2. educating old people and the general public about the changes in the social and physical environment which could promote better health in old age.

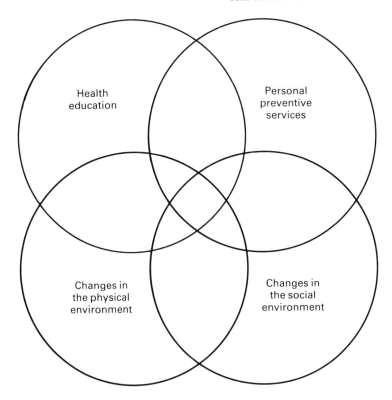

Fig. 1.9 The interrelated process of prevention

Personal preventive services

Every health and social service has a contribution to make to prevention in old age, but some are of particular importance:

Chiropody
General practice
Community nursing
Health visiting
Physiotherapy
Occupational therapy
Home helps
Social work
Income support services

However, it is essential for professionals to remember that the most important contribution to prevention in old age is made by old people themselves. Self-care is the most common and important type of care in old age. Professional care should be complementary to self-care and to the care given by family and friends.

These services are related to the other three means of prevention:
1. Health education is a personal preventive service.
2. Social changes, for example a change in public and professional attitudes towards older people, are essential if preventive services are to be organised and delivered with enthusiasm.
3. The development of well-designed easily accessible health centres in inner cities is of vital importance.

Changes in the physical environment

Older people would have fewer problems if their housing conditions were better, if public transport were more suited to their needs and if planners took the needs of older people fully into account when designing new towns and shopping centres.

1. Old people need education about ways they can improve their environment, for example by claiming a housing improvement grant.
2. The provision of advice from occupational therapists helps people with disabilities overcome the problems posed by the physical environment.
3. Changes in the social environment are often necessary, for example legislative changes, before improvements in the physical environment are brought about.

Changes in the social environment

Changes in the attitudes and beliefs of old people and of young people are essential if prevention is to the effective. Health education can only be effective in influencing individuals if it influences the beliefs and attitudes that prevail in society as a whole, and changes in the social environment expressed through changes in legislation bring about changes in the pattern of personal preventive services and in the physical environment. As in prevention at other ages, political change is often a necessary precursor before the means of prevention can be fully effective.

ETHICAL DILEMMAS

The prevention of disease bristles with just as many ethical problems as clinical medicine (Gray, 1979) and some are of particular relevance to prevention in old age.

The ethics of dabbling

It has been argued that many elderly people face such massive social problems because of their poverty that it is inappropriate and insensitive to try to influence aspects of their lifestyle such as their exercise patterns or diet. Two arguments are used to support this point of view. The first is that such an approach can lead to 'victim blaming', with the old person being made to feel totally responsible for all his or her problems, some of which stem from a lifetime of poverty and deprivation. Secondly, it has been argued that professionals should use their energy and influence to campaign for higher pensions and better social conditions for old people rather than expending it all directly on old people themselves.

However, in support of prevention it has been argued firstly that it could be seen as insulting form of paternalism if professionals were just to assume that elderly people should not be encouraged to consider the prevention of disease simply because they were poor and, secondly, the development of a preventive strategy and the application of pressure to improve pensions are not necessarily mutually exclusive.

The writing of this book indicates that the authors support the latter argument and accept that it is essential that well-paid professionals should recognise the importance of poverty and not simply concentrate on certain medical aspects of prevention.

The ethics of reframing

Before anyone will participate in any form of prevention, they have to accept that there is a problem. A difficulty encountered when working with older people is that the old person may not consider the problem to be serious. Sometimes he does not even consider that he faces 'a problem' or that he is 'at risk'. Before challenging the old person's view of his situation and attempting to change it, the possibility that this attitude might be valuable to the old person and essential to his mental wellbeing has to be considered.

In some people such attitudes are due to a mistaken belief, for example to the belief that all the problems of older people result from the ageing process or from 'God's will'. Such people will change their beliefs and attitudes when provided with accurate information. In other people, however, the attitude that 'I'm all right' is a means of coping with some of the anxieties and fears that they experience.

Common fears and anxieties alleviated by the attitude that 'I'm all right'

Fear of the future. The old person may prefer to focus on the present, and be reluctant to look ahead at the problems the professional would like her to consider.

Fear of failure. The old person may prefer not to try the preventive measures suggested because she is afraid she will try and fail, with subsequent damage to self-confidence.

Fear of disappointment. The old person may prefer to say 'I'm all right' rather than allow her hopes to be raised: most disabled old people have had enough disappointment from professionals to become cautious.

Fear of institutionalisation. The old person may fear that an admission of her problems or the fact that she is 'at risk' will lead to the suggestion that she should go into a home.

There are many other fears and anxieties which can alleviated by the steadfast attitude that 'I'm all right (Wilcock et al, 1982), and the doctor advocating prevention has to be aware that this attitude is not always due to ignorance. It may be of positive value to the old person, and the decision to challenge this attitude is an ethical decision and not simply an educational decision.

Important though it is to appreciate the ethical problems that occur in preventive medicine, it is equally important to emphasise that relatively few old people are forced to participate in preventive activities against their wish. Professionals still err on the side of caution and deny elderly people the right to accept or reject the challenge of health promotion. Elderly people certainly have a right to refuse preventive or therapeutic measures, but that right can only be competently exercised if elderly people are aware of the scope for prevention in old age and are adequately supported by sympathetic relatives and professionals if they do try to change their lifestyle and improve their health.

THE IMPACT OF PREVENTION

One effect of prevention is an increase the numbers of very elderly people in society, and there will therefore be an increase in the number of very elderly people suffering from those diseases that cannot be prevented, for example Alzheimer's disease. There has also been concern, however, that the prevalence of disabling disease, as opposed to the total numbers of people affected, will be increased by preventive activity, by encouraging the 'survival of the unfittest' (Isaacs et al, 1971).

There is an increase in the prevalence of certain disabling conditions due to an increase in the survival of affected individuals, for example in Parkinson's disease (Marsden & Parkes, 1977) and dementia (Christie, 1982), due to improvements in treatment and care. However, the possibility that we could be increasing the age-specific prevalence of disability is a worrying one, and the increasing incidence of fractured neck of femur is a worrying trend. There is, however, no evidence to suggest that the costs of prevention will outweigh the benefits, but there is a need for careful monitoring of the impact of preventive and therapeutic innovations by longitudinal studies of cohorts of elderly people. This is a type of research that is seriously underfunded.

REFERENCES

Adelstein A 1977 Mortality from tuberculosis: a generation effect. Population Trends 8, HMSO
American Association for Clinical Chemistry 1979 Aging, its chemistry. In: Proceedings of the Third Arnold O. Beckman Conference in Clinical Chemistry, Wishington
Busse E W, Maddox G L 1982 The Duke Longitudinal Studies of Normal Aging. Springer, New York.

Christie A B 1982 Changing patterns in mental illness in the elderly. British Journal of Psychiatry 140: 154–159
Fletcher C, Peto R, Tinker C, Speizer F E 1976 The natural history of chronic bronchitis. Oxford University Press, p45
Fries J M 1980 New England Journal of Medicine 303: 130–135
Gray J A M 1979 Man Against Disease. Oxford University Press
Isaacs B, Gunn J, McKechan A, McMillan I, Neville Y 1971 The concept of pre-death. Lancet 1: 1115–1118
Lewis A F 1981 Fracture of neck of the femur: changing incidence. British Medical Journal 2: 1217–1220
McKeown T 1979 The role of medicine. Blackwell, Oxford
Marsden C D, Parkes J D 1977 Success and problems of long-term levodopa therapy in Parkinson's disease. Lancet 1: 345–349
Rowntree S (ed) 1947 Old people: report of a survey committee on the problems of ageing. Oxford University Press
Schaie K W, Strother C R 1968 Psychological Bulletin 70: 671–680
Sheldon J H 1948 The social medicine of old age. Oxford University Press
Shephard R J 1978 physical activity and aging. Croom Helm, New York
Svanborg A, Bergstrom G, Mellstrom D 1982 Epidemiological studies on social and medical conditions of the elderly. EURO Reports and Studies 62. World Health Organisation, Copenhagen
United States Department of Health Education and Welfare 1979 Healthy people: the Surgeon General's report on health promotion and disease prevention. DHEW(PHS) Publication 79-55071. US Government Printing Office
Wilcock G K, Gray J A M, Pritchard P M M 1982 Geriatric problems in general practice. Oxford University Press
Wilson J M G, Jungner G 1968 Principles and practice of screening for disease. World Health Organisation, Geneva

2

Jeffrey Garland

Prevention of dependency

Dependency or trust in others, relying on them for support, is a complex concept which can be used in at least seven different senses. It can be universal or particular, acute or chronic, pertaining to an individual or a group, appropriate or inappropriate, condoned or condemned.

Inter-dependency

As part of being human, we accept inter-dependency, at least in theory. In fact, we may each generally contrive to live in a state of relative isolation breached only in times of unusual conviviality or extreme crisis. But at least for some of the time we depend on each other, whether for basic physical survival, or in a spiritual sense (as St. Paul said in Ephesians 4:25, we are 'members one of another').

Recognising inter-dependency helps the multi-disciplinary team work more productively with old people. The patient depends crucially upon the team. Members of the team — some more than others, or with less insight than others — depend on the patient to show recognition of the professional's need for a response to the treatment offered. Both sides are necessary for the equation of treatment, and it is important to appreciate this.

A developmental variable

Age-related dependency is a developmental variable. The human infant shows extremely high dependency in both physical and psychological functioning. Progress past developmental milestones sees a gradual lessening of dependency for the normal individual moving into adult life, although in Western culture the final transition to independence may not be clearly marked.

The picture presented by the severely impaired old person is described sometimes as 'second childhood'. One of the sharpest illustrations of this view is by Arnold Bennett (1910) depicting the oldest Sunday-school teacher, Mr Shushions, in Clayhanger:

The old man had lived too long; he had survived his dignity; he was now nothing but a bundle of capricious and obstinate instincts set in motion by ancient souvenirs remembered at hazard...He wore boots that were not a pair. His collar was only fastened with one button, behind; the ends oscillated like wings; he had forgotten to fasten them in front; he had forgotten the use of buttons on all his garments. He had grown down into a child again, but providence had not provided him with a nurse.

Providence, or rather the Health and Social Services together with the private sector, now provides carers, for survival needs at least. Hard-pressed staff in continuing care of the elderly comment: 'You keep them fed and clean, that's about all you have time for.' In the community, an old person's supporters in need of an evening out, unselfconsciously request 'someone to do a spot of babysitting'.

To view abnormal ageing in terms of regression to a state of childishness has an intuitive appeal when one considers how learned adult habits can be rapidly distorted in the process of accelerated ageing. However, the temptation should be resisted. It is facile to equate a malformed habit with an unformed one, and to view an old person as a 'child' who lacks potential for growth is to become an overprotective 'parent' whose care will smother any hint of independence.

Disadvantaged status

In sociological terms, dependency characterises the status of disadvantaged groups whose access to resources is unduly restricted. The 'structured dependency' of old people is tellingly described by Townsend (1981) who sees social policy as having created: the imposition, and acceptance of, earlier retirement; the legitimation of low income; the denial of rights to self-determination in institutions; and the construction of community services for recipients assumed to be predominantly passive. He comments: 'The routine of residential homes, made necessary by small staffs and economical administration, and committed to an ideology of 'care and attention' rather than the encouragement of self-help and self-management, seems to deprive many residents of the opportunity if not the incentive to occupy themselves and even of the means of communication.'

More than twenty years ago Townsend (1962) was making similar points about dependency, so it seems that little has changed in spite of a spate of research and the demands of pressure groups for higher pensions and more generous benefits, pensioner control of old people's homes, and health and housing improvements as rights rather than concessions.

Egalitarian views are not necessarily held by all who work with the elderly, but even those of us who see no real prospect of a significant reduction in the social disadvantage affecting many old people can recognise that the dependency inflicted by compulsory retirement, low income and paternalism has the associated risk of increased physical and psychological dependencies.

Even if we cannot reform society, we can take steps to ensure that patients and their supporters are informed of their rights, encouraged to exercise them, and if necessary are provided with an effective advocate.

A personality variable

Dependency has been described as a personality factor formed largely by early experience and operating in a relatively continuous and persistent way as a behavioural trait which may predict a degree of reliance on others in a given situation. A variety of terms, including 'group dependency', 'low self-efficacy', 'high need for affiliation' and 'low coping', have been used by different theorists.

To 'explain' an old person's behaviour by invoking a 'dependent' personality is circular and unhelpful, promoting therapeutic nihilism. It is more constructive to view dependent behaviour in terms of social learning theory, and to bear in mind that, as behaviour is a function of personality and environment, a treatment setting which selectively rewards progress in independence can promote the learning of independent behaviour even in a patient who has a long history of finding reliance on others rewarding.

A phenomenon of therapy

Psychotherapists have described acute dependency as a phenomenon of the therapeutic relationship, consisting of a marked degree of reliance by the patient on the therapist's authority and prestige. Goldfarb & Turner (1953) report that with elderly patients this factor can be used with particular advantage by the therapist cautiously and selectively assuming a position of dependency in relation to the patient, whose self-confidence is much enhanced if this is done judiciously.

Dependency of this nature often appears in geriatric medicine, where most of us have seen patients in rehabilitation arise and walk at the request of consultant and white-coated retinue at a ward round, to the amazement and chagrin of ward staff who have been struggling, but without success, to encourage the patient to walk.

An acute dependency reaction may appear in hospitalisation of a patient, young or old. It may also characterise behaviour of a staff group, producing undue deference in meetings with team members of high status, or excessive help-seeking in a situation which does not require it, such as summoning a duty doctor in the early hours of the morning to a continuing care ward immediately after the long-expected natural death of an elderly patient.

While resenting the negative aspects of such dependency, medical leadership can unwittingly foster them, and this is perhaps a particular risk for the more charismatic and energetic geriatrician who understandably lacks time to reflect on the psychological consequences of his behaviour.

Reduced activities of daily living

In medical and nursing care of the elderly, dependency is usually understood as a reduced ability to perform the activities of daily living. Accident, illness, the physical, psychological and social changes of ageing, may all be involved in increasing an individual's dependency to a critical extent, so that hospitalisation is required.

As Mulligan (1973) explains, classifying patient according to degree of dependency into a small number of care groups (usually three: high, intermediate and low dependency), facilitates hospital planning, the organisation of progressive patient care, the monitoring of patient progress and the measurement of workload.

Levels of dependency (cognitive and/or behavioural) may also be used either in the community or in an institution to predict an old person's ability to cope with a particular environment. An example of this approach is offered by the widely-used Clifton Assessment Procedures for the Elderly (CAPE) of Pattie & Gilleard (1979) which translates raw scores into five levels ranging from 'independent' through to 'maximum dependency'.

While such measurement is desirable and has many useful functions, serious problems, both theoretical and applied, impede our ability to understand and assess impaired activity. For example, a general decline in intellectual functioning with ageing has been widely reported, as Botwinick (1978) confirms, but the nature and extent of this decline is a matter of controversy.

Schaie (1974) has maintained that there is no universal decline, pointing out that investigators frequently have failed to take account of increased cautiousness of older subjects confronting inappropriately designed problem-solving tasks which smack of the schoolroom. In subsequent publications he has been one of a growing number of researchers who contend that reliable decrement for *all* intellectual abilities and *all* subjects cannot be found until the late eighties.

Cross-sectional studies comparing different age groups at the same point in time tend to overestimate 'normal' decrement in intelligence with ageing, as inferior education and health experience of members of the older cohorts tend to be given disproportionate influence.

On the other hand, longitudinal studies following a group through from early or middle life to late life appear to underestimate 'normal' decrement for a variety of reasons, of which the most prominent appear to be a tendency for selective survival in the more intelligent subjects, with relatively higher attrition of the less intelligent.

Features of these two approaches are combined in the cross-sequential method which is being employed in several ongoing large-scale studies of intellectual changes with ageing, and effectively uses the strengths of both cross-sectional and longditudinal approaches while largely limiting their liabilities to error. An effective brief introduction to the complex topic of age differences and age changes is offered by Chown (1983).

Among the problems of an applied character which beset our understanding of the nature of intellectual and other dependencies in old people is the abundance of assessment methods that have been used. Many of these are 'one-shot' tests, making it very difficult to compare findings across various studies. Some have only 'faith' validity to recommend them, that is to say they are used persistently without proper scrutiny. An example is the serial sevens subtraction test, sequentially subtracting 7, beginning with 100. Smith (1967) found that, in a sample of 132 normal subjects aged 18–65, only 56 completed the task successfully, and many produced error patterns that literal interpretation of the test's results would have suggested to be highly sinister. Yet this test (together with many others of questionable value) remains in use.

Psychologists should not be too critical of the prevalence of ramshackle do-it-yourself assessments of dependency in the elderly, since, with relatively few exceptions, there is a surprising lack of ecologically valid and psychometrically well-founded psychological assessment techniques in this area. However, work on the development of such techniques is in progress in a number of centres in this country and we can expect the next five years to see major advances.

Perhaps the central aspect of the practice of geriatric medicine is the reduction of treatable dependency and the maintenance of effort towards improved understanding and management of dependency not currently treatable. Because dependency can be multiply determined, not only by accident, illness, physical, psychological and social changes with ageing, but also by the patient's environment and idiosyncratic reaction to being ill and requiring help, a seventh and final form of dependency, which will be the focus of the remainder of this chapter, needs to be distinguished.

Excess disability

Brody et al (1971) and other investigators have described excess disability in the aged as difficulty in functioning that exceeds expectations based on a patient's physical condition alone. The consultant or other team member who notes that a particular elderly patient is not making the progress in rehabilitation which would be expected normally, given her physical status, and begins to speculate that the patient 'lacks motivation', may be observing this phenomenon. The visitor to a continuing-care geriatric area, surveying the scene with fresh eyes, is also likely to note excess disability in a setting in which patients' needs as individuals must often be subordinated to the demands of nursing routines.

It is generally the grosser forms of excess disability that demand attention. Almost without exception, across a variety of settings, all elderly patients 'could do better' in the sense that their functioning ability does not consistently match their physical potential.

'Institutionalism' — behaviour problems deriving from the nature of a hospital setting and independent of whatever difficulties a patient had before entering — has been described by Wing & Brown (1970), outlining the clinical picture presented by many chronic schizophrenics in long-stay areas, as one of docile submissiveness, with the patients inactive and unresponsive.

A similar debilitating environment appears to affect some old people in institutional care. It involves reduced self-confidence, increased psychological dependence and decreased physical ability. We lack objective normative standards for evaluating the appropriateness of this form of dependency in a given elderly patient: much of our reaction is likely to be highly subjective, as we project our own expectations on to the patient, so that the indolent care staff member is content to let patients doze in their chairs, while her lively colleague drags everyone to their feet to fling bean bags.

The institutional environmental features which contribute to increased dependency for the elderly patient have been described by George & Bearon (1980). They include: lack of privacy, considerable social distance between staff and patients, structured rules enforced by staff with arbitrary discipline imposed for infringements, a large part of each day spent in 'block treatment' by all patients sharing the same activity, lack of occupational resources, lack of variation in daily routine, and relative isolation from the community.

In geriatric medicine the patient's physical needs come first, and resources for meeting psychological or social needs are extremely limited, so the preceding catalogue of institutional incentives to dependent behaviour in the elderly should be seen in perspective.

It must be recognised, too, that meeting dependency needs appropriately is essential in order to promote independence. Necessary supports must be built into any rehabilitation programme, and a degree of dependency is an appropriate reaction for any patient. As Stotland (1969) points out:

> The patient enters hospital with at least a minimum of expectation that one of the goals of the hospital as an institution is to help patients ... If the hospital staff does not have confidence in itself or is not motivated strongly toward their joint goal, it would be delusional for the patient to assume that the staff could has few guideposts. Furthermore he lacks the confidence to evaluate the guideposts that he does find. He must depend on the staff for an evaluation of the prospects for their joint enterprise.

While appreciating that the patient's position is essentially a dependent one, it is important to appreciate the institutional pressures that maintain unnecessary dependency. One of the more useful contributions to a growing body of evidence is by Barton et al (1980), who describe in a controlled observational study how help-seeking behaviour in elderly nursing-home residents is promoted. In the context of early morning washing and dressing it was noted that dependent behaviour by residents was followed immediately and continuously by supportive behaviour from carers, while independent behaviour by residents had no social consequences at all.

If some dependence appears to be learned through positive encouragement, can independent behaviour be learned in its place by manipulating the consequences of behaviour, the environmental contingencies? Barton's co-workers are currently following up this possibility for the behaviour which they observed. For many other types of behaviour by elderly patients, which will be described shortly, it has already been established that dependency can be reduced by increased selectiveness in responding by others in the patient's environment.

A worthwhile note of caution concerning the modification of old people's excess dependent behaviour is sounded by Rebok & Hoyer (1977). They remind us that the linkages between the old person, her behaviour and the physical and social setting are complex. Institutions are geared to deal with the average patient rather than with the eccentricities of the abnormally dependent individual. The significance of reverse behaviour change is still not well understood by the would-be behaviour modifier who can be the target of subtle shaping by the elderly patient, supporters or care staff who decline to cooperate or, in excess of zeal, over-cooperate.

Moreover, as Kastenbaum (1964) explains, the presentation of dependent behaviour is complicated by the 'crisis of explanation' linked with the onset of old age. When late life is encountered as if unexpected, the result for some old people is that they do not do much or plan much, because they literally do not know what has happened to them, cannot explain to themselves where they are or who they are, and cannot determine in which direction to move and for what purpose.

Kalish (1969) indicates that the impact and predictive significance of increased dependency with the onset of late life is likely to show wide individual variations, and Roth (1972), commenting on the stronger relationship between chronic physical illness and affective disorder in elderly *males* suggests that for the ageing male physical disability has more powerful psychological implications.

Almost certainly, gerontologists were formerly too ready to assume that institutional admission *per se* necessarily increases dependency in old people. Many of the supposed ill-effects are difficult, if not impossible, to disentangle from the deterioration in functioning which frequently precipitates admission. Moreover, the effects of a major move of any kind in late life, irrespective of direction, can disrupt independent behaviour.

A number of commentators have underlined cultural differences in the way in which independence for old people is viewed that distinguish, for example, the United Kingdom and the United States. In this country, it has been suggested, we recognise the right of an old person to autonomy, but we do not frame a corresponding obligation upon the old person to exercise that right. In the United States, however, the right and its attendant obligation are linked by cultural expectation, with consequently a more negative attitude towards, and less provision for, the wilfully dependent.

PREVENTION OF DEPENDENCY

How may we persuade elderly patients who show dependency of this kind that they should want to be more autonomous? And how do we work productively with their helpers and supporters to promote an environment that increasingly encourages independence?

The answers can be grouped under seven headings: improved service delivery, more effective and unified assessment procedures, specific use of individual and family therapy, development of cognitive training methods, implementation of findings from behaviour modification, milieu therapy and provision of prosthetic environments.

These possibilities will be discussed in turn, primarily in relation to dependency in the form of excess disability, while recognising that the boundary between this and legitimate dependency can be extremely difficult to define. We must also bear in mind that for any given patient dependency in other senses may also confine their ability, and that not all forms of dependency can, or should, be 'cured'.

Improved service delivery

In *The Last Refuge* (1962) Townsend decided: 'The general conclusion of this book is that communal homes of the kind which exist in England and Wales today do not adequately meet the physical, psychological and social needs of the elderly people living in them, and that alternative services and living arrangements should quickly take their place'. The residents are still waiting for this revolution, but quiet changes in the climate of residential care of the elderly are taking place. Norman's *Rights and Risk* (1980) is perhaps the best-known of a number of recent publications to argue the case for maintaining independence of living, as far as possible, within residential care.

A more clarion call to geriatric departments came from Stewart with *My Brother's Keeper?* (1971), whose innovative use of 'reablists' at the Edgware General Hospital is widely known, although, for a variety of reasons, not widely imitated (in my experience).

It is widely agreed that, if old people are to be more independent, professionals providing services need to change from a 'do-gooding' attitude to a more open approach, enabling and even encouraging recipients to voice criticism if they wish.

The principle of normalisation in the delivery of service (Wolfensberger, 1972), by which the recipient is encouraged as far as possible to function in an environment that approximates to normal, and in which the prospect of functioning closer to maximum potential is enhanced, appears to be advancing into geriatric services. Bromley (1978) clearly recognises this in his suggestions for remedying the aversiveness in appearance and behaviour that locks many elderly patients into a cycle of dependency. Not uncommonly they show decreased mobility, spontaneity and responsiveness as indicated by posture, gesture, facial expression and eye contact, and this, Bromley points out, produces difficulty in social interaction for supporters and carers, who lack feedback, feel they are not getting through, and tend to limit contact, withdrawing the personalised support that can encourage independent activity by the patient.

Bromley's suggestions for possible remedies include: more effective education on ageing for supporters and carers and empathy training for these groups, more attention to grooming and cosmetic care for elderly patients, self-help and social skills training for patients, and an improved quality of life in institutions to facilitate patients' social contacts.

As Brody (1977) indicates, the hospital offering continuing care for the elderly is significant in a number of respects: it represents to older people and their families a possible future; by maintaining therapeutic optimism it can demonstrate that patients' functioning can improve; a social planning function can be met by studying the paths of new admissions and finding where community services are lacking; the hospital has a pivotal role in exploring problems, referring them to more appropriate resources, mobilising social services to avoid or delay admission; it is a base for community services to operate from; and it is a site for training, research and educational programmes.

Inevitably, geriatric services based on hospitals are adopting with increasing certainty the minimal intervention approach (Kahn, 1975), which is least disruptive of the old person's usual functioning in her usual setting (unless there is imminent risk of acute medical problems).

However, it is virtually impossible for the geriatrician not to get drawn into the social welfare issues which are prominent in the lives of so many elderly patients. One reason for this, as Chapman (1979) shows, is that elderly people's access to social services is frequently restricted by: poor publicity of services, proliferation of services and benefits, complicated application procedures, control and rationing by officials, and reluctance to apply.

If social services can be remote from the needs of elderly clients, hospital-based health services for the elderly have no room for complacency. Cohen (1980), reviewing mental health services for the elderly in the United States, finds them to be largely passive, with limited outreach and little education in the community about the facilities they offer. Accessibility relates to availability, visibility, appeal and readiness to deliver, Cohen comments, and asks sardonically whether a would-be filmgoer would buy a cinema ticket if she was unable to find out what film was showing, or any meaningful details of cast, cost, times of showing, or critics' reviews.

Similar reservations could be raised concerning the accessibility of geriatric and psychogeriatric services in this country, although (and perhaps this is a cultural difference) the issue as stated by Cohen does not appear to cause overmuch concern in the United Kingdom.

Another issue which has received relatively little attention in this country is the risk to independence which precipitate delivery of community-based services to the elderly can entail. Blenkner et al (1971) report a four-year study of elderly people receiving comprehensive social services, compared with a group of similar need but without services, and note that the former group showed increased dependency and higher death rates.

The long-term effects of community support which in the short term appear to reduce dependency and avert hospital admission are still emerging. For example, in Oxford where a joint-funded project to provide home care seven days a week for 'at risk' elderly has postponed hospitalisation in the short-term for a number of its clients, in the long-term a number of clients are likely to age at home with this degree of continued support until they reach such high dependency that any option of Part III admission could be blocked, leaving continuing care in hospital as the only solution. As the scheme is being carefully monitored, it is expected that this outcome will not be a regular occurrence, but the need of careful liaison to reduce risk of ultimately increasing dependency for such clients is clear.

A major obstacle to improved accessibility of services is that providers, already extremely busy, fear they will be overwhelmed. Such fears emerged rapidly in Oxford during a recent multi-disciplinary review of diminishing numbers and lack of fresh faces in groups for supporters of elderly people seeking counselling, information and the opportunity to share feelings. A research study to investigate the position and to evaluate new groups or a more attractive alternative was proposed but is still in the balance, amidst fears in some quarters that 'we might be overwhelmed' by demand from supporters for a more accessible and appealing product.

Perhaps in relating service delivery to the reduction of dependency, we need above all to be more consistent in strategies of applied research: selecting among possible interventions, developing these, choosing when interventions should take place and monitoring the effectiveness of the chosen intervention. All interventions are experiments, but in clinical practice it is rare for them to be carefully controlled, with the goal of repeating those which on balance appear to increase independence and discontinuing those followed by increased dependency.

Attempts to measure the output of services by progress towards stated objectives are, as Wright (1974) illustrates, of challenging complexity, and it is not surprising that attempts to relate service delivery unequivocally to the reduction of dependency are rare.

Effective and unified assessment

There is lack of uniformity between studies of similar populations of elderly people dependent in terms of activities of daily living, and it is highly unusual to find a group of separate studies which actually use the same measure of dependency. Although there are many local assessment procedures in different parts of the United Kingdom, none that I have seen links directly to available service resources, so the professional who usually oversees completion of the assessment together with the patient, her supporters or helpers, is likely to work mechanically through the procedure, seeing little relevance in the exercise.

A number of promising procedures have been developed, for example CARE (Gurland et al, 1977), but no one approach has yet found general favour. Without a shared language to describe the degree of dependency and change in dependency following intervention, research comparing the effectiveness of different treatment approaches cannot be properly carried out and significant progress is unlikely.

Dependency in terms of excess disability is even more problematic to assess. The route to its better understanding, I suggest, is through pinpointing specific problems and direct observation of behaviour which incorporates not only the help-seeking actions, but also their antecedents and consequences. For example, when assessing excess shouting for assistance by a bedfast patient in a geriatric ward, valuable data can be gathered from a tape recorder left by the bed, with the agreement of the patient and the care team. Fitted with a time-switch, this device will record, say, for five minutes every one or two hours throughout the desired period and yield data that can be discussed with the patient (if co-operative) and care staff, not only to assess the problem, but also, as all worthwhile clinical assessment should do, to point to possible solutions.

Hearing such tapes means appreciating directly that staff typically do not respond to such patients when they are being quiet, but reward them with *intermittent* attention (powerful in maintaining behaviour) when they begin to be noisy. If this relationship is established, a wide variety of options can be systematically applied to reduce the frequency of excess shouting. (Noisemaking which is maintained by inadvertent reinforcement is of course only one form of noise-making and this assessment approach will not be relevant for *all* noisy patients.)

While assessment instruments are becoming more sophisticated, we have to remember that people, not instruments, make the decisions on acceptable levels of dependency. Carstairs & Morrison (1971) and many subsequent researchers find that 'Part III acceptability', for example, shows marked variations in the restrictiveness with which it is interpreted by different homes.

Individual and family therapy

From a psychodynamic standpoint, psychotherapy for the elderly is seen by Verwoerdt (1981) as a worthwhile enterprise which has the reduction of dependency as one of its major goals. Sherman (1981) offers perhaps the most substantial description to date of the value of individual counselling for the client who needs to overcome the demoralisation attendant on the inevitable losses and changes of ageing.

In cognitive therapy, the patient is helped to identify and distinguish characteristic patterns of thinking which are productive or destructive, is supported in developing patterns of thought related to positive coping and in trying out environmental changes and modes of behaviour consistent with these. This type of therapy has been reported by Hussian (1981) to be effective in assisting the elderly resident (depressed by admission to residential care) to cope by practising such thoughts as 'This place is home now and I'm going to make the most of it' and 'If I feel a low spell coming on I'm going to fight it by keeping my mind active.'

Cognitive therapy deals effectively with relatively complex chains of thought as well as with the simple statements above. For example, an 81-year-old patient living alone became increasingly depressed because her son in Canada had not written to her for some months. Enquiry revealed that her last letter to him had ended with the phrase 'don't come to my funeral' which *for her* conveyed 'please come and see me soon, please don't wait until you have to come to my funeral because then it will be too late'. The task of disentangling this misinterpretation and restarting correspondence was facilitated for me by the techniques of this therapeutic approach.

A wide-ranging literature supports the value of individual therapy for enhancing independence in old people, and recent references to problem-solving groups which can involve the elderly and focus on patients developing their own decision-making skills hold promise. Rose (1977) introduces this approach very clearly.

Information and counselling for supporters of dependent old people is an expensive resource, and the most appropriate first line of approach is to direct their attention to self-help information on access to resources and the reduction of dependency. This can be gained most economically from one of the popular texts aimed at supporters in need of advice. Such manuals, whether British (Gray & McKenzie, 1980) or American (Mace & Rabins, 1981), offer immediate practical hints on coping and the availability of aids, while encouraging their readers to preserve as far as possible an independent lifestyle for the old person.

Eyde & Rich (1983) propose that families function as informal case managers, record-keepers, information repositories and most importantly as providers ensuring continuity of care. They can help the old person to sense belonging; integrate past, present and future; and adapt and adjust to changing demands.

These authors submit that families, as the crucial agent of observation and response to change in a dependent elderly member, need to be supported by professionals rather than supplanted by caseworkers eager to impose their values and standards of care. They caution, however, that the pattern of support offered by the family tends all too often to be reactive rather than proactive. The old person may become progressively more disturbed and disturbing, but she and the family 'don't want to bother' outsiders, and day-to-day interaction within the family can be too limited to produce useful communication about possible solutions to their dilemma.

From my observation, collusion by supporters with the very dependency that concerns them is not uncommon. A worried woman whose 75-year-old father lived with her told me that he was 'going crazy' and pressed for his hospitalisation. Asked for an example of this 'crazy' behaviour, she replied: 'That's easy! The other day he came down from his room at two o'clock in the afternoon and asked for breakfast. Breakfast! He must be going mad.'

'And what did you do?' I asked.

'Oh, I gave him breakfast.'

I was silent.

'Didn't I do the right thing?'

'Well, could you have done anything else?'

'I suppose I could have said, "Look, Dad, it's two o'clock in the afternoon. If you want food you can have something, but it's too late for breakfast."'

'Would it have *cured* him?'

'Probably not, but it would have helped him to realise that there's a right time for breakfast and he can't have it any time he fancies!'

Exchanges of this sort can be frequent when communicating with supporters who have been humouring an old person, often because they have been driven into doing so by persistent demands. In the short term, humouring may ease a situation, but in the long term it is likely to produce further problems. However, the supporter tempted by short-term gains of peace and quiet may need exceptional personal qualities and counselling support in order to maintain a long-term strategy.

The solutions which families can produce to contain the dependency of an elderly member can be inspired and far superior to anything a professional could come up with. But sometimes the solution is apt to contain the seeds of future problems, as was the case with a supporters' group member who proudly told me that she had solved the problem of her elderly mother's nocturnal wandering. In common with the rest of the group I leaned forward, eager to hear of this breakthrough.

'In the end, it was quite simple. I've moved my bed into her room and I'm sleeping across the threshold. She can't wander now.'

'I see...And how does your husband feel about this?'

'What do you mean, how does he feel?'

'Has he said anything about this idea?'

'No, not really. In fact, he's gone rather quiet lately...'

Nobody laughed. Disturbed nights, as Sandford (1975) reports, are one of the most significant features in reducing supporters' ability to cope with an old person's dependency (together with mental impairment and incontinence). Families supporting an elderly member who is mentally ill tend to be discriminated against in the deployment of statutory domiciliary services, it has been suggested, and it is not uncommon for the lonely struggle of supporters to produce unthinking collusion and desperate remedies.

Cognitive training

There is increasing interest in training approaches which enable a dependent old person to use intellectual ability more effectively.

Reality orientation (Holden & Woods, 1982) can be applied both in intensive individual or small-group 'classroom' sessions and in the form of '24-hour RO' as a consistent practice in all contacts with the old person. The process involves sharing information, prompting and cueing recognition and repetition of key facts, sensory stimulation, labelling the environment in a clear and attractive way to promote orientation, and praising in a natural and positive way all responses that indicate alertness and attempts to use information correctly.

While many helpers and supporters use the elements of this approach to a considerable extent, it is rare for it to be used consistently without training, and even trained staff can find RO difficult to maintain because it demands considerable dedication and patience. It is not effective with highly dependent patients, and gains in intellectual functioning from RO tend to disappear if the programme is discontinued.

For those in close contact with old people, the approach is of special value in offering a framework for building purposeful communication which is more rewarding for both sides than the half-hearted random interaction which is more usually found.

Memory training of a more intensive kind for old people has been explored in a number of recent research studies, and Zarit et al (1982) suggest that its potential may usefully be explored even in severe memory loss associated with brain failure. The aim of memory training is to promote relatively intact skills and to help the patient use alternative strategies if appropriate. Techniques which have been studied include: practice on memory tasks in individual or group sessions; progressively stretching by gradual increments the length of time over which memory is required; attention training; use of external aids such as signposts and route following, colour-coding, use of diary and/or notebook, alarms or other cues to prompt recall; use of internal aids such as visual imagery to build face–name associations or identify places needing association with items to be remembered.

Much of this work is translated from the field of rehabilitation of brain-injured patients, and its value for the dependent elderly is actively being explored. From the literature it is widely accepted (Botwinick, 1978) that old people's performance on cognitive tasks can be improved if they are instructed in mediational techniques such as the use of mnemonic devices and encouraged to use these. Note-writing is an obvious example of an everyday aid to integrate material and aid recall, but its use by the dependent elderly has not been investigated systematically, perhaps because of the widespread impression that old people cannot make use of notes, see no reason for using them and often find them indecipherable even to themselves.

Denney (1979) finds that, while older subjects are usually poorer in performance on problem-solving tasks, short-term training in general produces improvement, although some experimental interventions designed to improve functioning have actually had negative effects. A major problem in interpreting research in this field, she suggests, is that nearly all studies use group means, although it is probably the case that some individuals within any group of old people benefit from intervention, while others do not.

The degree of intellectual impairment is perhaps the most obvious factor in determining susceptibility to intervention, but anxiety level could be an important variable. Only a few studies, with inconclusive results to date, have made some preliminary efforts to couple anxiety management training with problem-solving performance.

Behaviour modification

This method of reducing dependency, which is widely used with most patient populations, begins with the premise that much human behaviour is learned and operates on an individual's environment to produce consequences. If the consequences of an act are valued by the individual concerned, the behaviour is likely to be reinforced so that it becomes more liable to recur and become part of the person's repertoire. If the consequences of an act are not those desired or valued by the person, that behaviour becomes more likely to change and less liable to repetition.

As is the case with reality orientation, many helpers and supporters practise an approximation to the approach without formally labelling it, and indeed behaviour modification in a crude sense is an experience of everyday life.

As Hoyer (1973) explains, the way in which ageing is conceptualised determines to a great extent the character of intervention to reduce dependency. If helplessness, excessive demands for attention and other dependencies are attributed to 'senility' or 'dementia', they will not be seen as subject to potential change. In practice it will not be possible to implement the consistent programme of positive reinforcement of independent behaviour (providing a consequence valued by the old person and contingent on independent action), and extinction of dependent behaviour (not providing the attention which has come to be associated with dependency), if such problems are viewed as wholly the result of 'old age' which cannot be treated.

The literature on the application of behaviour modification to dependency in late life is substantial and many techniques have been found to be effective in increasing independence even in institutionalised patients. One of the better short reviews of progress in this extremely important area is by Hussian (1984).

Among the activities of daily living which have been successfully modified in the elderly are washing, personal grooming and hygiene, mobility, improved continence, reinstatement of acceptable eating habits, social activity and communication and participation in recreational activity.

The period of observation which is an essential prerequisite of behaviour modification usually is revealing, not only of the patient's behaviour, but also of the responses of those around her, some of whom may well be unwittingly maintaining the problem by their responses.

During baseline observation of 'Agnes', a geriatric patient who had been attacking fellow patients, hitting them and inflicting 'Chinese burns', it became evident that the attacks generated at least nine different responses from care staff: scolding, ignoring, separating the antagonists, distracting her attention, secluding her, forcing her to apologise to the victim, slapping her lightly on the wrist with the injunction 'see how you like it!', avoiding the situation by leaving the room, and even sitting Agnes down for tea and sympathy and asking her reasons for attacking others (these in the classic delinquent response were usually given as 'I don't know' followed by 'I won't do it again'.)

While the hitting may well have been intrinsically rewarding for Agnes, it is likely that some staff responses were more rewarding than others for her, since from her general behaviour she clearly valued staff attention and used to follow nurses round like a little dog. Intermittently her attacks won her attention — even an angry response may be more attractive than no response at all, for it was noteworthy that during baseline observation when she was not attacking others she was totally ignored.

Testing this theory involved agreeing on a standard response to all attacks: to say 'No, Agnes' immediately, separate her from her victim without comment, and retire. At the same time staff members were asked to approach her when she was not hitting people and to spend a little time with her then, immediately withdrawing if she showed any sign of hitting. Within one week of this change, her 'strike rate' was down by 70 per cent, although even within this first week some staff members found it most difficult to modify their own behaviour and tended to revert to preferred patterns.

Milieu therapy

Modification of a hospital's environment in a planned way is a tool for increasing independence of elderly patients, and Denham (1983) has collected essays on improving the quality of life for the long-stay patient which effectively address the most important issues.

Such planned changes, which have been widely evaluated for their impact on patient dependency, range from the relatively minimal (deployment of a few student volunteers for a limited time) to detailed and expensive innovations deploying extra resources, trained staff, or major changes in the layout of wards and increased input of occupational therapy and activity programmes.

These are generally reported to have encouraging immediate results, but *any* change in a work setting may do this, and proper evaluation is hampered when one examines most of these studies because of their imprecise measurements, frequent lack of controls, confusion over objectives and lack of long-term follow-up. This is unfortunate, because the factor of *environmental docility* for the elderly (Lawton & Simon, 1968), indicating that as competence decreases external environmental factors become progressively more important in determining behaviour, is well documented. Lawton's review (1979) of therapeutic environments for the elderly indicates the distance that many institutions still have to travel.

Prosthetic environments

In a much-quoted paper, Lindsley (1964) discussed the needs of 'geriatric behavioural prosthetics' – hospitals or homes which offer multiple sense–modality displays, fail–safe devices in OT, response–force amplifiers, and a wide range of technology to facilitate independent functioning and to relieve patients' 'terminal boredom'.

The prosthetic environment, as Lawton (1970) points out, has to offer: the capacity to provide basic life maintenance, functional health provisions, support for perceptual and cognitive behaviour, assistance in physical self-maintenance, assistance in instrumental self-maintenance, support for the patient's personal effectiveness and facilitation of social functioning. Having offered this imposing list, Lawton goes on to propose that for some of these factors there is for the elderly person no place like home, the most prosthetic environment of all.

It is necessary to remember that dependency in the sense of excess disability can be exacerbated by the complex and conflicting expectations which the old person, health or social services, and society, have of each other.

The role of a hospital patient carries not only exemptions but also obligations to want to get well and to co-operate with treatment. The role of a resident of a continuing-care setting may appear to be exempt from responsibility, without corresponding obligations. Reciprocity of effort is more likely to be characteristic with a patient who is aware of receiving treatment than with a resident in continuing care who is not normally expected to demonstrate progress in rehabilitation. As an 83-year-old resident of a continuing care ward put it when I asked her opinion of being in hospital: 'Hospital? I'm not in a *hospital*, because nothing is being done to me here. I'm in a sort of general hotel where they take in all the overflow from the main hospital!'

Awareness by an old person that payment is being made, whether for 'treatment' or for 'care', may act as a disincentive for independent effort. It can be observed that some old people in both hospital and in social services accommodation are apt to point out to staff who encourage independence: '*You've* paid to do that', or to complain 'I've paid my stamps all my life' or 'I've sold my house to come here!' However, it should be noted that other old people do not cite financial reasons for any economy of effort on their part, even when they may know they are paying more than others for the service they get. Furthermore, some of those who do cite a payment factor in defence of excess disability may well be rationalising. However, the role of a paid carer who at the same time is expected to encourage the recipient of care to exercise independence is not easy to interpret, and the resultant difficulties cannot be dismissed as unimportant.

Some old people are indeed vulnerable during independent action, but it can be argued that, as the dividing line between normal safety precautions and an excessive preoccupation with risk avoidance is not always clear, providers of services, understandably concerned that accidents could produce adverse reaction and even legal consequences, consistently tend to err on the side of caution. Acceptable levels of risk, underwritten by the authority of senior service providers, need to be defined and advanced to public acceptance, but this is a delicate issue and progress may well be slow.

CONCLUSION

I have suggested that there are many different forms of dependency, that agreement is lacking on how we should best interpret and assess the most medically relevant of these, and that there are many approaches which can be used to maintain and enhance the elderly patient's independent functioning.

Within geriatric medicine understanding of this polymorphous concept will remain unreliable in the absence of a widely used, unified, multidisciplinary method of asessment of dependency in terms of reduced functioning in the activities of daily living, and incorporating a more objective understanding of the manifestations of excess disability. Such a development would not make the problems of geriatric medicine go away, but it would promote the effective planning and evaluation necessary for a truly accountable service responsive to patients' needs.

REFERENCES

Barton E M, Baltes M M, Orzbech M J 1980 On the etiology of dependence in older nursing home residents during early morning sessions: The role of staff behaviour. Journal of Personality and Social Psychology 38: 423–433

Bennett A 1910 Clayhanger. Penguin Books, Harmondsworth, Middlessex

Blenkner M, Bloom M, Neilson M 1971 A research and demonstration project of protective services. Social Casework 52: 483–499

Botwinick J 1978 Aging and behavior. A comprehensive integration of research findings, 2nd edn. Springer, New York

Brody E M 1977 Long-term care of older people. A practical guide. Human Sciences Press, New York

Brody E M Kleban M H, Lawton M P, Silverman H A 1971 Excess disabilities of mentally impaired aged: impact of individualized treatment. The Gerontologist 11: 124–133

Bromley D B 1978 Approaches to the study of personality changes in adult life and old age. In: Isaacs A D, Post F (eds) Studies in geriatric psychiatry. Wiley, Chichester, ch 2, p17–40

Carstairs V, Morrison M 1971 The elderly in residential care. Report of a survey of homes and residents. Scottish Health Service Studies No. 19, Scottish Home and Health Department

Chapman P 1979 Unmet needs and the delivery of care. A study of the utilisation of social services by old people. National Council of Social Service, Bedford Square Press, London

Chown S M 1983 Age differences and age changes. In: Nicholson J, Foss B (eds) Psychology survey no. 4. The British Psychological Society. Leicester, ch 3, p 62–87

Cohen G D 1980 Prospects for mental health and aging. In: Birren J E, Sloane R B (eds) Handbook of mental health and aging. Prentice-Hall, Englewood Cliffs, New Jersey, ch 41, p 971–993

Denham M J (ed) 1983 Care of the long-stay elderly patient. Croom Helm, London

Denney N W 1979 Problem solving in later adulthood: intervention research. In: Baltes P B, Brim O G (eds) Lifespan development and behaviour, vol 2. Academic Press, New York

Eyde D R, Rich J A 1983 Psychological distress in aging. A family management model. Aspen, Rockville, Maryland
George L K, Bearon L B 1980 Quality of life in older persons. Meaning and measurement. Human Sciences Press, New York
Goldfarb A I, Turner H 1953 Psychotherapy of aged persons. American Journal of Psychiatry 109: 116–121
Gray M, McKenzie H 1980 Take care of your elderly relative. Allen & Unwin/Beaconsfield, London
Gurland B, Kuriansky J, Sharpe L, Simon R, Stiller P, Birkett P 1977 The comprehensive assessment and referral evaluation (CARE): Rationale, development and reliability. International Journal of Aging and Human Development 8:9–42
Holden U P, Woods R T 1982 Reality orientation psychological approaches to the 'confused' elderly. Churchill Livingstone, Edinburgh
Hoyer W J 1973 Application of operant techniques to the modification of elderly behaviour. The Gerontologist 13: 18–22
Hussian R A 1981 Geriatric psychology. A behavioral perspective. Van Nostrand Reinhold, New York
Hussian R A 1984 Behavioral Geriatrics. In Hersen M, Eisler R M, Miller P M (eds). Progress in Behavior Modification, Vol. 16 p 159–183. Academic Press, New York
Kahn R L 1975 The mental health system and the future aged. The Gerontologist 15: 24–31
Kalish R A (ed) 1969 The dependencies of old people. Occasional Papers in Gerontology, No. 6, Ann Arbor, Michigan: The University of Michigan, Wayne State University Institute of Gerontology
Kastenbaum R (ed) 1964 New thoughts on old age. Springer, New York
Lawton M P 1970 Assessment, integration and environments for older people. The Gerontologist 10: 38–46
Lawton M P 1979 Therapeutic environments for the aged. In: Canter D, Canter S (eds) Designing for therapeutic environments. A review of research. Wiley, Chichester, p 233–276
Lawton M P, Simon B 1968 The ecology of social relationships in housing for the elderly. The Gerontologist 8: 108–115
Lindsley O R 1964 Geriatric behavioral prosthetics. In Kastenbaum R (ed) New thoughts on old age. Springer, New York
Mace N L, Rabins P V 1981 The 36-hour day. A family guide to caring for persons with Alzheimer's Disease, related dementing illnesses, and memory loss in later life. The Johns Hopkins University Press, Baltimore
Mulligan B 1974 Measurement of patient–nurse dependency and work-load index. King's Fund project paper, London
Norman A 1980 Rights and risk. A discussion document on civil liberty in old age. National Corporation for the Care of Old People, London
Pattie A H, Gilleard C J 1979 Manual of the Clifton Assessment Procedures for the Elderly (CAPE). Hodder & Stoughton, Sevenoaks
Rebok G W, Hoyer W J 1977 The functional context of elderly behavior. The Gerontologist 17: 27–34
Rose S D 1977 Group therapy. a behavioral approach. Prentice-Hall, Englewood Cliffs, New Jersey
Roth M 1972 Recent progress in the psychiatry of old age and its bearings on certain problems of identity in earlier life. Biological Psychiatry 5: 103–125
Sandford R A 1975 Tolerance of debility in elderly dependents by supporters at home: its significance for hospital practice. British Medical Journal 3: 471–473
Schaie K W 1974 Translations in gerontology: From lab to life: intellectual functioning. American Psychologist 29: 802–807
Sherman E 1981 Counseling the aging. An integrative approach. Free Press, New York
Smith A 1967 The serial sevens subtractions test. Archives of Neurology 17: 78–80
Stewart M 1971 My brother's keeper?, 2nd edn. Health Horizon, London.
Stotland E 1969 The psychology of hope. Jossey-Bass, San Francisco
Townsend P 1962 The last refuge. Routledge and Kegan Paul, London
Townsend P 1981 The structured dependency of the elderly: a creation of social policy in the twentieth century. Ageing and Society 1: 5–28
Verwoerdt A 1981 Psychotherapy for the elderly. In: Arie T (ed) Health care of the elderly. Essays in old age medicine, psychiatry and services. Croom Helm, London

Wing J K, Brown G W 1970 Institutionalism and schizophrenia. Cambridge University Press, Cambridge.
Wolfensberger W 1972 The principle of normalization in human services. Leonard Crainford National Institute of Mental Retardation, Toronto
Wright K G 1974 Alternative measures of the output of social programmes: the elderly. In: Culyer A J (ed) Economic policies and social goals: aspects of public choice. Martin Robinson, London
Zarit S H, Zarit J M, Reever K E 1982 Memory training for severe memory loss: effects on senile dementia. The Gerontologist 22: 373–377

3

J. A. Muir Gray

The prevention of family breakdown

INTRODUCTION

The belief that the modern family does not care as well for its elders as families formerly did is widely held and commonly expressed in both popular and professional writing. This is not a new belief. It has been expressed for at least a hundred and fifty years. The Report of the Royal Commissioners on the Poor Law in 1834, for example, stated that 'the duty of supporting parents and children in old age or infirmity is so strongly enforced by our natural feelings that it is well performed even among savages, and almost always so in a nation deserving the name of civilised. We believe that England is the only European country in which it is neglected.' Seventy-five years later, in 1909, the next Royal Commission on the Poor Laws reiterated the complaint that there was a 'disinclination of relatives to help one another' and emphasised 'that there is not the same disposition to assist one another that there was years ago'. This belief is one aspect of a more general belief, namely the belief that life in general was better for old people in the past (Gray & Wilcock, 1981; Moroney, 1976).

Increasingly, however, historical evidence suggests that both beliefs are wrong. Elderly people were not more highly valued by society or by their families in times past. In fact, the opposite appears to have been the case. Poor old people who were no longer able to continue working were so little valued by society that they were offered no pension and had to depend largely on their children if they wished to live at home. The latter were, however, often unable to offer help because they too were also poor. and the old people were therefore often forced to enter the workhouse. Rich old people were obviously able to maintain their independence, but they often did so by maintaining control over their estates and businesses so tightly that their own children were kept dependent on them. The children kept in subjugation often became resentful, and a vicious cycle developed. The longer the elderly parent continued to hold the reins, the more resentful the grown-up children became, and the more afraid grew the old person as to what might happen to him if he were to be so unwise as to relinquish control of the family's resources, with the result that he held on even more tightly and suspiciously.

The spectre of King Lear haunted the imagination of many a rich old person (Thomas, 1976). The introduction of old age pensions and the acceptance of the need for retirement, even in small family businesses such as farms, have reduced the tensions and improved family relationships. Furthermore, when comparing the modern family with its precursor, it is essential to take into account a number of social and demographic changes which make it more difficult for relatives to provide support even if they are willing to do so (Table 3.1)

Furthermore, many elderly people, particularly elderly women, have no living relatives, in part because of the impact of World War 1 on the cohorts that are elderly today.

It is important to emphasise that, although this chapter refers to the problems faced by families and elderly people in developed countries, the same types of problems are found in many developing countries and are becoming more common and more serious as urbanisation breaks up the traditional pattern of society much more quickly than occurred in the developed world (Ssenkoloto, 1982).

THE NATURAL HISTORY OF FAMILY BREAKDOWN

All relatives, whether families or single sons and daughters, who look after an elderly relative have a breaking point, a point at which family tension becomes intolerable. Some families are much more tolerant than others, and one of the most important factors which determines the point at which a relative will feel she cannot carry on is the nature of the relationship between the old person and the person who is principally involved in caring. Not all old people are nice old people. Some are unrewarding to care for: self-centred, demanding and manipulative. These characteristics are not the result of ageing, being almost always traits that have been present for many years. Often the 90-year-old who dominates her 50-year-old daughter will have dominated her throughout her whole life.

If the old person was a generous, unselfish parent when her children were young, they will be more tolerant when he becomes dependent on them than if he has always been self-centred and selfish, but even a family in which there have always been good relationships can reach breaking point. However, the better the relationship, the longer will the family be able to cope and

Table 3.1 Relevant Trends In Family Structure

Decreasing trends	Increasing trends
Family size	Population mobility
The proportion of daughters who remain spinsters	Women working
	Marital breakdown and remarriage
The age at which people marry	

the longer will they take to reach breaking point. Paradoxically, those families in which relationships have not been good and who therefore need more help may receive less help because they irritate those from whom they seek it by appearing to be uncaring. This is, in part, due to the fact that they are often ashamed to admit their dislike of, or hostility to, their elderly parent and in part due to the fact that the old person who is so unpleasant at home to her unmarried daughter may appear pleasant and cooperative to her general practitioner and district nurse.

There are three common types of change which precipitate a breakdown in the family support by increasing family tension to breaking point.
1. The cumulative effect of chronic disabilities (Fig. 3.1).
2. The effect of an acute illness or a series of acute illnesses affecting the old person (Fig. 3.2).
3. The effect of problems affecting the principal carer, for example physical exhaustion or illness, or a social problem not directly related to the old person, for example redundancy affecting either herself or some other member of the family (Fig. 3.3).

Chronic deterioration of the old person

The assessment of the elderly person who is suffering from a chronic decline in functional ability is no different whether the old person is living with relatives or living alone. There are, however, certain symptoms which have been shown to be particularly difficult for families. Some of them are obvious; others may apperar insignificant to the person who does not have to live with them all day (Table 3.2).

It is important to emphasise that even an apparently insignificant trait, for example the way the old person drinks his tea or the noise he makes with his false teeth, can become intensely irritating to the relatives who live with that old person. With this type of problem the dependency of the old person gradually increases as his ability decreases, and the tension in the family gradually builds up. Only rarely, however, does the family reach breaking point solely because of the gradual deterioration of the old person's condition. Almost always there is a precipitating factor, either an acute illness of the old person or the onset or aggravation of a problem affecting those who care for him.

Acute illness

An acute illness by itself is rarely sufficient to cause a breakdown in the system of support given by relatives. More frequently an acute illness is either the 'last straw', either because it is the cause of a sudden increase in the dependency of the old person or because it leads to a hospital admission for the management of the acute illness, with the result that the family are provided with the opportunity of appreciating just how severe their burden

FAMILY BREAKDOWN PREVENTION 41

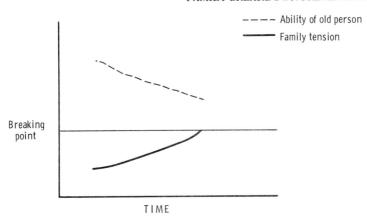

Fig. 3.1 Natural history of family breakdown. Gradual increase in tension due to gradual increase in ability of old person

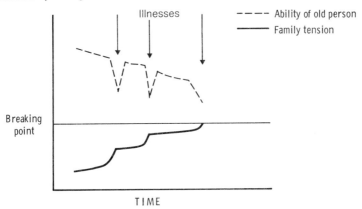

Fig. 3.2 Natural history of family breakdown. Stepped increase in family tension caused by a series of acute illnesses

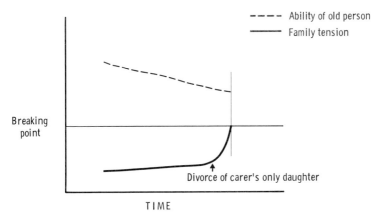

Fig. 3.3 Natural history of family breakdown. Increase in family tension caused by divorce of carer's only daughter; no significant change in ability

Table 3.2 Checklist of symptoms most difficult for relatives to bear

---
Faecal incontinence
Urinary incontinence
Wandering at night and disturbing the relatives' sleep
'Risky behaviour', for example with matches or with the gas or refusal to use adequate heating, both because of the anxiety generated and because of the feeling that the old person cannot be left alone
Unsavoury table manners
Repetitive behaviour
Repetitive speech
Inability to respond to other members of the family
Heavy physical dependency
Antisocial behaviour

Sandford (1975)

has been and how pleasant life is without their elderly relative. In the latter type of case the breakdown in family support is manifested by refusal of relatives to cooperate in arranging the discharge of the old person from hospital. In such cases it is the decrease in family tension which is the crucial factor.

Problems of the principal carer

Within the network of people caring for an elderly person, one of them can usually be identified as the principal carer, the one who does most for the elderly person, and it sometimes happens that it is a change in the condition or situation of the carer that prompts not only the referral of the old person but also the presentation of the old person as the principal cause of the carer's problem.

The principal carer who is the member of a supportive family is obviously able to cope with personal problems for longer than the carer who has an unsupportive family, or the single carer. Single sons and daughters face particularly difficult problems when coping with disabled elderly relatives (Table 3.3).

When the old person lives with a whole family and not with a single carer, he may be the cause of problems within that family. However, he may be affected by, and even blamed for, problems for which he is in no way responsible (Table 3.4).

It is important to remember that any strain on the family, even though it has nothing directly to do with the old person, may lead to a call on the doctor to 'do something', by which is usually meant finding a long-stay bed.

THE SCOPE FOR PREVENTION

Having defined the problems that lead to family breakdown, it is tempting to assume that the development of services which prevent or alleviate these

Table 3.3 Checklist of main points in assessment of the principal carer

Common problems	Special problems for single carers
1. Physical disease; many carers are themselves middle-aged	The single carer may not have anyone to notice a change in her health status and encourage her to consult her GP
2. Physical exhaustion	The single carer has no-one with whom to share the physical or psychological burden
3. Depression	Particularly common among single daughters who have given up a career to care
4. Anxiety	Related to the uncertainty about what will happen after the death of the old person
5. Financial problems	Most serious when single carer is not working
6. Housing problems	The single carer may be at risk of homelessness when the old person dies

Table 3.4 Checklist of problems experienced by families looking after an elderly relative but which are not necessarily caused by the elderly relative

1. Inability to go out because it is felt that the old person cannot be left alone; often the fears on which this reluctance are based are groundless
2. Inability to entertain visitors because it is believed that they will be embarrassed
3. Problems with teenage children; although these are rarely caused by the old person directly, overcrowding can aggravate quarrels with and between teenagers
4. Marital problems; usually aggravated rather than caused by the presence of an elderly relative
5. Financial problems

particular problems will prevent family breakdown. On *prima facie* grounds the case for believing this is sound, but there have been too few intervention studies to allow this conclusion to be drawn from firm evidence. The reason for the lack of evidence is that the methodological problems involved in studying such problems are considerable: for example, little is known about the natural history of family breakdown, and the selection of controls poses serious technical and ethical problems. Research workers have therfore not yet organised a study which could have demonstrated the effectiveness, or ineffectiveness, of different types of intervention. Most studies have been descriptive, with the research workers making deductions about the types of intervention they believe to be the most effective on the basis of their observations. These reservations must be borne in mind when reading the following section, but it is also important to bear in mind that the development of services for the relatives supporting old people should not be left until conclusive proof of effectiveness has been obtained. The benefit offered by many of the services that will be described is so obvious that a randomised trial would be unethical.

The many different interventions that are considered to be effective means

Table 3.5 Checklist of main points for discussion with a family and an old person who wish to live together

1. The need for some meals to be taken separately, for example one meal a day
2. The need for each side to have a few evenings apart and the ability to entertain alone
3. The benefits of whole days apart, for example once a month
4. The benefits of separate holidays
5. The need for a clear agreement about money, which will probably need to be reviewed after 6 months

of preventing family breakdown may be classified in two ways. Firstly, they may be classified with respect to the objective of intervention. Alternatively, the interventions may be classified by their timing, as primary, secondary or tertiary.

Classification by the timing of the intervention

Primary prevention

There are four ways by which primary prevention of family breakdown may be achieved, although the feasibility of primary prevention is limited because the crucial decisions are often made before a professional has been consulted.

Prevention of an unwise move. Too often the main cause of a family's problem is that the elderly person moved too soon from his own home to live with his relatives. This may happen after an acute illness, when relatives may say, 'You should't live alone any more', or after a bereavement when relatives sometimes relieve their own anxieties by telling the old person she should 'Come and live with us', an offer which may be accepted by the old person too distressed to weigh up the options rationally. Such offers are often made, and accepted impulsively without adequate discussion and reflection only to be regretted later by which time it is often impossible to reverse the situation, usually because the old person's house has been sold or relinquished.

In other cases a younger relative, most commonly a single daughter, moves in to live with her elderly parent under pressure from her siblings. Fortunately, fewer doctors now put moral pressure on single daughters by making statements such as, 'Your mother shouldn't be left on her own now', but it is easy to give the impression that this is the case and thus put pressure on a single daughter to give up her house and her job and move in with her mother or, more commonly, to reinforce the pressure already being exerted by married siblings and their spouses.

In general the ability of an elderly person to cope safely on his own is greatly underestimated by anxious relatives; too often the decision that an old person should give up her home is made too quickly and too early, but if doctors and other health professionals are involved with families at such times, they are in a good position to counsel caution.

Prevention of overcrowding. One persisting myth is that it was customary for three generations of a family to live in the same dwelling. This was not the universal custom and, whenever possible, the old person would live *near* but not *with* her family. Nowadays elderly people often move to live with relatives, and the overcrowding that results contributes significantly to family tension and therefore to the ability of the younger relatives to cope. An elderly relative moving in to live with a couple with two teenagers in a three-bedroomed semi-detached house can cause significant overcrowding of both sleeping and living space, but even where physical overcrowding is not a problem the benefits of both the old person and her family having their own territory make it preferable for each to have their own dwelling, either a separate dwelling or a granny flat. Unfortunately this is not always possible, but if the old person has enough money, perhaps from the sale of a house, the family should be advised to look at the possibility of buying a suitable dwelling near at hand in preference to house-sharing.

In the United Kingdom an elderly council tenant has the right to apply to the local authority in which his children live for a transfer under the National Mobility Scheme, but in practice most local authorities are able to rehouse only a small proportion of those elders who wish to move. Nevertheless, a general practitioner's letter stating the medical reasons why a move is desirable should be offered as it will often have some influence (Rossiter & Wicks, 1983).

More elderly council tenants are helped to move by housing associations, and for elderly private tenants this is often the only way to move to another part of the country. Housing associations build similar dwellings at similar rents to local authority dwellings but, because they are not controlled by local councils, they are not restricted to the rehousing of local people. Relatives should be advised to ask their local housing department for the names and addresses of all the housing associations for elderly people in their neighbourhood and to apply directly to them. As with local authorities, a doctor's letter is usually influential but will not automatically ensure rehousing.

Promotion of good relationships. When an old person goes to live with relatives, there may be an initial 'honeymoon' period followed by the development of tension due in part to the fact that the two parts of the three-generation family are living without the type of ground rules that most families develop; not surprisingly, because such ground rules usually develop over a period of years. They are with one another too much, every meal, every evening, every weekend, and even though both the old person and his younger relatives wish to have more privacy, neither side may wish to suggest it for fear that they night be thought to be ungrateful, or rejecting, respectively.

It is often easier for an outsider to make simple suggestions such as the proposal that the old person should always have one meal a day in her room than for a relative to do so, and it is therefore possible for a doctor or nurse to prevent the souring of relationships by giving advice on a few common points of potential friction when the move is being discussed or arranged (Table 3.5).

Provision of information. Relatives need information not only about the help that is available but also information about the need to seek help early if the old person is deteriorating, or if they feel the strain of caring is increasing for any reason.

Secondary prevention

The most effective and efficient way for a busy primary care team to practise secondary prevention is to makes use of the contacts with the team initiated by the old person or by her relatives; to use what has been called the opportunistic approach. The basis of this approach is that when any member of the extended family consults, the opportunity is used to enquire if any problems or difficulties are developing.

Practices with an age/sex register can complement this approach by using the register to identify those families which have not made contact in the course of the preceding year and by visiting them when one member of the team is in their neighbourhood and has time to visit.

Tertiary prevention

The more effective the management of established problems, the longer will relatives continue to support the old person.

Classification by objective

Any measure that prevents a decline in functional ability or quality of life of an old person will postpone the breakdown of his informal support system. The prevention of problems in old age therefore indirectly helps the supporters of old people. In this chapter, however, I will discuss those services that have as their main objective the prevention of family breakdown.

The prevention of physical tiredness

Those looking after disabled elderly relatives not infrequently become very tired. Usually the fatigue is the result of number of different strains, but there are two problems which contribute significantly to the development of physical fatigue — onerous domestic duties and broken sleep.

Measures which can reduce the burden borne by families include the provision of domiciliary nursing to relieve relatives from the need to bathe the elderly person, the provision of help with the laundering of soiled linen and clothes, and the provision of help with household tasks, such as cleaning and shopping, although it is sometimes more valuable to the carer to have someone stay with the old person to that she can go shopping herself, than to have someone else shop while she stays at home with the old person as she does for the rest of the twenty-four hours.

Broken sleep is a major problem. It is caused by either disturbance by the old person during the night, or anxiety, or both. Measures to prevent broken sleep are of two types. Firstly, there are those which have as their objective the prevention of disturbance, which includes all measures necessary to improve the depth and duration of the old person's sleep, for example day care, the introduction of a calm evening routine which promotes sleep, and, if such measures fail, the prescription of hypnotics. Secondly, there are measures which can minimise the disturbance even if the old person wakes, for example the provision of a commode in the bedroom for the old person who needs help to reach the toilet in the middle of the night.

The anxiety of the caring relative is usually reduced if these measures prove to be effective. If they are ineffective, or if the carer remains so anxious that she is unable to sleep well even though the elderly person is sleeping more soundly, the admission of the old person to a home or hospital for a short stay to allow the carer a few nights of undisturbed sleep is an effective means of ensuring sleep and therefore of preventing the breakdown of support.

Prevention of social problems

There are two ways in which the contribution of relatives can be costed. One way is to put a financial value on the suffering of relatives. This is obviously difficult to do precisely, but such a costing is essential in any valid cost–benefit analysis. A simpler method of costing is to calculate the opportunity cost of caring by calculating the financial consequences for the caring relative if she were to use the hours she spends caring in some other activity, for example in paid employment. This is of particular relevance for the single son, or more usually, daughter who has given up work to look after an elderly parent. For this group of people financial assistance is essential, and in recognition of this the United Kingdom government introduced the Invalid Care Allowance in 1976 for carers of working age who were not in paid employment. This is not an adequate substitute for lost earnings — in 1981 it was equivalent to only 19 per cent of the gross average weekly earnings for full-time female workers (Equal Opportunities Commission, 1982a) — but it brought some relief, particularly as the allowance carries with it a contribution to the National Insurance Fund, which entitles the carer to a pension as though she were working.

Many carers, particularly single daughters, also have housing problems. The single child looking after an elderly parent who is a council tenant may have to leave the dwelling in which she has lived, her home even if it was not her tenancy, after her parent's death. Similarly, the single child of an elderly owner–occupier may lose her home unless the parent's will leaves the dwelling to her alone.

These problems impose extra strains on carers, and their prevention by enlightened policies prolongs the carer's ability to look after the elderly relative.

The prevention of stress

In this context the term 'stress' is used to describe the effects that the strains of caring for a disabled elderly person have on the carer's physical and mental wellbeing. Stress is obviously relieved by relieving strain, so all the measures described in the previous sections of this chapter are important means of preventing stress, but there are interventions which can directly prevent stress even if they do not affect the strains.

Simply by listening to the relatives' complaints the professional can relieve stress, particularly if he is able to help the carer to express any anger of bitterness she may feel. Many relatives feel very guilty about their angry thoughts but are unwilling to express them to others because they are afraid that they will be thought to be uncaring. The comfort given by the assurance that feelings of anger and a desire to hit the old person are common reactions to strain and that they do not indicate that the relatives are uncaring is often considerable. The type of intervention may be called counselling, to distinguish it from family therapy. The latter technique involves the whole family and has as its objective the resolution of the fundamental causes of that family's tensions, whereas the objective of counselling is only to relieve the stress that such tensions cause. It is often helpful to bring together all members of the family in an attempt to help both the old person and her younger relatives to express their feelings, but the difficulties of changing family tensions that have been established for decades should not be underestimated, and this type of intervention should only be attempted by those who have had special training in psychotherapeutic techniques.

THE IMPORTANCE OF STYLE

Important though it is to use effective methods for relieving strain and stress, the style of intervention, the way in which help is given, is also of vital importance in the prevention of family breakdown, as one recent study demanstrated.

The characteristic of professional intervention that relatives deemed to be most important was technical competence. They were not simply seeking sympathy and support but useful advice from skilled professionals. If, however, the intervention was delivered in a particular way, relatives were

more effectively supported than they would have been had the only contribution of the professional been his technical expertise. The characteristics of good professional practice defind by relatives were displayed by professionals if they:
1. arranged interviews promptly
2. made it clear who they were, where they came from and why they were visiting
3. showed sensitivity in their dealings with the elderly persons
4. were willing to listen to the supporters and showed concern about their wellbeing
5. gave clear explanations
6. understood the possible causes of confusion
7. where a diagnosis of dementia was made, through careful questioning, established the precise problems which its management posed
8. agreed a clear and promptly implemented plan of action
(Levin et al, 1983)

A sensitive, as well as a competent, response to a request for help is therefore one important characteristic of effective intervention. The other important characteristic is a planned approach to the family's problems. If the professionals not only respond to the present problem sympathetically but also institute a plan for shared care, the anxiety felt by relatives can be considerably diminished. If, for example, the family are assured that they will receive two weeks' relief every eight weeks, no matter how ill, or well, their elder may be, they will suffer much less stress than if they are offered only an indefinite promise of help at some unspecified time.

Only shared care can be successful care, and if family breakdown is to be prevented, the relatives have to feel that they are not only members of the caring team, but its most important members.

It is also essential for government policies to take into account not only the actual contribution that family support can and could make but also the aspirations and expectations of relatives (Finch & Groves, 1980). Care must be taken that emphasis on community care and praise for the virtues of the family are not simply used as a means of shifting the burden of caring from the statutory services to the relatives of elderly people, most often to their daughters, for they may have other aspirations (Equal Opportunities Commission, 1982 b). It is a matter of regret for both professionals and society as a whole if relatives neglect their elders, but it is equally regrettable if relatives are exploited by professionals and society

Acknowledgement

The ideas in this chapter were developed in discussion with Gert Almind, Charles Freer and Gregg Warshaw, with whom I worked on the Kellogg Foundation's Study Group on the family doctor's contribution to medical care in old age (Kellogg, 1983).

REFERENCES

Equal Opportunities Commission 1982a Caring for the elderly and handicapped
Equal Opportunities Commission 1982b Who cares for the carers?
Finch J, Groves D 1980 Community care and the family: a case for equal opportunities. Journal of Social Policy 4: 487–511
Gray J A M, Wilcock G K 1981 Our elders. Oxford University Press
Kellogg International Scholarship Program on Health and Aging (1983) The contribution of the primary care doctor to the medical care of the elderly in the community. Kellogg Foundation
Levin E, Sinclair I, Gorbach P 1983 The supporters of confused elderly persons at home. National Institute for Social Work, London
Moroney, R M 1976 The family and the state. Longman, Harlow
Rossiter C, Wicks M 1983 Crisis or challenge: family care, elderly people and social policy. Study Commission on the Family
Sanford J R A 1975 Tolerance of debility in elderly dependents by relatives at home. British Medital Journal 3: 471–473
Ssenkoloto G M 1982 Family support for the elderly. World Health: May 22–25
Thomas K V 1976 Age and authority in early modern England. Proceedings of the British Academy, vol 62

4 J. A. Muir Gray, G. Almind, C. Freer and G. Warshaw

Screening and case finding

THE SCOPE FOR SECONDARY PREVENTION

Ludwig Wittgenstein pointed out that many differences of opinion can be resolved by clarifying the meaning of the terms that are being used in the debate, for while so doing it often becomes apparent that those who believe that their views are in conflict find that they are locked in conflict because each is using a certain term in his own way, with his own particular meaning, without ever having asked the other person what he means when he uses that term. This has been the case with secondary prevention.

This term was defined by the World Health Organisation as being 'all measures designed to reduce the prevalence of a disease in a population by shortening its course and duration' (Hogarth, 1978), but this term became less popular as two more precise terms — screening and case-finding — became more popular.

The coining of these terms was based on two assumptions. The first was that the natural history of many diseases passed through three stages:
1. Asymptomatic
2. Symptomatic, but unreported to the health services
3. Symptomatic and reported.

The second assumption was that earlier intervention would improve outcome. On these assumptions it was argued that an aim of preventive services should be to detect asymptomatic disease and, if that was not possible or practicable, to encourage earlier reporting and detection of symptomatic disease. The former strategy was termed 'screening', the latter 'case-finding', but the meaning of these terms has also changed in recent years.

Precise definitions were suggested by the World Health Organisation in a classic Public Health Paper, 'Principles and Practice of Screening for Disease', published in 1968 (Wilson & Jungner, 1968), although the definitions they proposed were long established, having been coined by the Commission on Chronic Illness in 1951 (Commission on Chronic Illness, 1957). The WHO definition of screening was 'the presumptive identification of unrecognised disease or defect by the application of tests, examinations or other procedures which can be applied rapidly. Screening tests sort out apparently well persons who probably have a disease from those who probably do not'. This elegant definition has stood the test of time, as was to be expected, for the term 'screening' was not a neologism: the first recorded use of the term 'screen', cited in the Shorter Oxford English Dictionary, in 1573, was to describe an apparatus for 'the sifting of grain, coal, etc.' and the choice of the term was particularly appropriate, for the objective of screening tests is to separate the wheat from the chaff. The term 'case-finding', in contrast, was used to describe the detection of established disease which had not previously been reported to health professionals.

The original distinction between screening and case-finding was, therefore, made on the basis of the natural history of disease. More recently, however, another criterion has been used for deciding whether an intervention was screening or case-finding, and this criterion depends on the person who initiates the contact at which the intervention takes place. If the contact has been initiated by a doctor or health worker the activity was said to be screening, whether the doctor is testing for asymptomatic disease or enquiring about unreported problems. If, on the other hand, the search for hidden problems takes place at a contact initiated by a member of the public, the activity, whether it be the search for asymptomatic disease or the enquiry about problems other than the one that was the original reason for self-referral, was called case-finding. The difference between the two sets of meaning can be summarised diagrammatically (Tables 4.1 and 4.2).

Table 4.1 WHO distinction, made with respect to the timing of the intervention

Type of contact	Stage in natural history	Asymptomatic	Symptomatic but unreported
Doctor-initiated contact		Screening	Case-finding
Patient-initiated contact		Screening	Case-finding

Table 4.2 Unofficial, but popular, use of the terms, with the distinction based primarily upon the person initiating contact

Type of contact	Stage of disease	Asymptomatic	Symptomatic
Doctor-initiated contact		Screening	Screening
Patient-initiated contact		Case-finding	Case-finding

In some ways these differences are academic, since the early detection of asymptomatic disease or undeclared health problems is important whichever definitions are used — but it does help to understand the literature, since many authors seem either unaware of these different usages or do not state their precise definitions.

SCREENING IN OLD AGE

The belief that disease should be sought at an asymptomatic stage became popular in the early 1960s when medicine was more confident than it is today. There was a rapid growth in the number of screening tests believed to be effective, and multiphasic screening, the application of a number of screening tests, became popular. In the late 1960s, however, the publication of two important reviews of screening — the WHO paper (Wilson & Jungner, 1968) and a collection of eassays published by the Nuffield Provincial Hospitals Trust (Cohen, Williams & McLachlan, 1968) — poured cold water on the uncritical enthusiasm for screening that had hitherto prevailed. In these reviews, criteria against which screening procedures should be tested were listed and the application of those criteria, which were more rigorous than many of those used previously, revealed that some of the screening tests which had been introduced, or which were being proposed, by enthusiastic advocates could not considered to be of proven value. The criteria were:

1. The condition sought should be an important health problem.
2. There should be an accepted treatment for patients with recognised disease.
3. Facilities for diagnosis and treatment should be available.
4. There should be a recognisable latent or asymptomatic stage.
5. There should be suitable tests which were both sensitive, namely able to detect all of the cases, and specific, namely unlikely to diagnose anyone who did not have the disease as being a sufferer.
6. The test should be acceptable to the population.
7. The natural history of the condition, including development from latent to declared disease, should be adequately understood.
8. There should be an agreed policy on whom to treat as patients.
9. The cost (including diagnosis and treatment of patients diagnosed) should be economically balanced in relation to possible expenditure on medical care as a whole.
10. Screening should be a continuing process and not a 'once and for all' project.

The Nuffield Provincial Hospitals Trust review also included a very useful scheme for the evaluation of screening procedures:

    A. *Definition of the problem*
    1. What abnormality of medical significance is to be predicted or detected?
    2. What prevention or therapy is to be offered?
    3. Which group(s) is to be screened?

4. At what stage(s) is detection aimed?
5. What investigation and tests are proposed?

B. *Review of position before screening*
1. Evidence concerning the prevalence, natural history and medical significance of the abnormality, with conclusions on the adequacy of the evidence.
2. Evidence concerning effectiveness of previous methods of preventing the disease.
3. Evidence concerning the effectiveness of previous methods of treating the disease.

C. *Review of evidence concerning the screening procedure*
1. Evidence concerning the effectiveness of the proposed diagnostic method(s).
   a. Applicability to group whose investigation is proposed
   b. Error rates, positive and negative
   c. comparison with traditional diagnostic methods
   d. Availability of resources
   e. Applicability
   f. Cost
   g. Conclusions on state of evidence on diagnostic method.
2. Evidence concerning the effectiveness of the proposed treatemt.
   a. Applicability to group proposed
   b. Comparison of effectiveness with treatment following conventional diagnosis
   c. Availability of resources
   d. Acceptability
   e. Cost
   f. Conclusions on state of evidence on treatment.

D. *Conclusions concerning the state of evidence on the problem as a whole*
1. Synthesis of evidence concerning the natural history of the disease and the effects of the screening procedure as a whole, diagnosis and treatment being considered together
2. Listing of medical gains and losses and comparison with similar balance sheets for alternative approaches to the problem
3. Listing of financial costs and gains and comparison with alternative approaches.

E. *Proposals for acquisition of further evidence*
Is further evidence necessary, and if so, what? What are the logistics of the proposals and their relationship to available resources?

F. *Proposals for initial applications*
What application is justified? For what design, scale, and duration should it be planned? How should it be supervised, and what resources should be committed? Is the proposal mainly as a service on a research basis and, if the latter, what information, or technical or operational developments, should be pursued?

These criteria have, however, been interpreted differently in different countries. In the United Kingdom, screening procedures are divided into two categories — those which satisfy these criteria and which should therefore be delivered to the total at risk population as part of the National Health Service, and those which do not satisfy the criteria. The latter should continue to be the subject of research, with any persons offered the relevant tests clearly informed that they are being offered a test that is not of proven benefit as part of a research project.

In Canada, a different classification was proposed by a task force convened to report on the periodic health examination. The task force gave five classes of recommendation for screening (Canadian Ministry of National Health and Welfare, 1979):

> After assessment of the evidence regarding each condition by means of these sets of criteria, five classes of recommendations were developed as follows:
> A. There is good evidence to support the recommendation that the condition be specifically considered in a periodic health examination.
> B. There is fair evidence to support the recommendation that the condition be specifically considered in a periodic health examination.
> C. There is poor evidence regarding the inclusion (or exclusion) of the condition in a periodic health examination, and recommendations may be on other grounds.
> D. There is fair evidence to support the recommendation that the condition be excluded from consideration in a periodic health examination.
> E. There is good evidence to support the recommendation that the condition be excluded from consideration in a periodic health examination.

This categorisation was further complicated by the introduction of a system of grading for the effectiveness of the treatments of those identified by the screening; the treatments being classified as either Grade I or Grade II, and by the introduction of six criteria to be used when considering tests in Group C.

Although this system has some advantages over the British system, it also has its weaknesses, principally that the doctor or health planner considering a test has to base his decisions on whether or not to include it in his services on imprecise terms such as 'good', 'fair' and 'poor'.

In the past twenty years a number of different screening tests have been proposed for use in elderly populations (Table 4.3).

There is as yet no evidence that any of the tests in Table 4.3 is useful in shortening the duration of any disease, or in the prevention of a loss of functional ability or in preventing the need for long-stay care if applied to a whole population of elderly people. These tests are often useful if there is a

Table 4.3 Tests suggested as being useful for the early detection of asymptomatic disease in old age

Chest X-ray
Urea and electrolytes
Haemoglobin
Erythrocyte sedimentation rate
Whole blood count
Culture of midstream urine specimen
Urinalysis
Thyroid status
Faecal occult blood
Tonometry

clear clinical indication or a clinical suspicion that a problem perceived by the old person or his supporters may be caused by a disease that can be diagnosed by one of these tests, but there is no indication for their routine use in healthy old age.

In general, North Americans are more enthusiastic about screening than people working in the United Kingdom, the difference in behaviour being due in part to the different systems of medical remuneration, for periodic health examinations have an obvious attraction for a medical profession that receives payment for each item of service. However, the difference is not simply due to financial factors: there is a real difference in attitude towards intervention between the two cultures, for there was also a long-standing genuine enthusiasm for the periodic examination of adults in the United States (Charap, 1981), which also had an important financial dimension, because the principal proponent — Dr. E. Fisk — worked in the 'Life Extension Institute' which was open to policy-holders of Metropolitan Life and other insurance companies.

Generalisations about North America have, of course, to be made with considerable caution because there are differences of opinion within it. Nevertheless, the approach to screening of asymptomatic disease in old age is more aggressive in North America. The guidelines produced by the American College of Physicians suggest that breast, rectal and pelvic examinations, mammography, the testing of stool for occult blood, and the measurement of blood pressure are validated screening procedures for people over the age of sixty-five (American College of Physicians, 1981). These tests were also recommended by the Institute of Medicine (Fielding, 1979) and endorsed by the American Medical Association, albeit with words of caution (American Medical Association, 1983). None of these would be regarded as being of proven efficacy in the United Kingdom.

CASE-FINDING IN OLD AGE

Screening is the search for asymptomatic disease; case-finding is the search for unreported problems, and a number of studies have demonstrated that elderly people have many unreported problems (Williamson et al, 1964). Before discussing case-finding, however, it is essential to define the natural history of a problem in old age, for the term 'problem' is used so often that its meaning is no longer the same to all who use it. To the professional, a problem is a situation or condition that poses an appropriate challenge to his skills; to an old person a problem is a difficulty, but not necessarily a difficulty for which professional help should be sought.

A number of stages in the evolution of a problem can be identified:
1. Development of the causal condition or situation.
2. The old person experiences difficulty in some aspect of his life.
3. Discussion with relatives and friends.
4. The old person decides that the difficulty is one that is appropriate to

bring to the attention of a professional.
5. Contact is made with the professional.

If the old person simply cannot make contact with the appropriate professional, either because he is immobile or because he has difficulty in communicating, case-finding, namely the identification of the unreported problem, will be of benefit to the old person. It will not necessarily solve his problem, either because the problem is insoluble or because there are insufficient resources to solve his problem and the old person may be disappointed, but his problem will have been brought to the attention of the appropriate professional, as the elderly person wished. There are no ethical problems in the detection of problems at stage 4 of their evolution. The identification of problems at stage 2 can, however, pose ethical dilemmas.

If the reason that the old person does not think professional intervention necessary is ignorance, the professional has an obvious duty to point out to the old person that the difficulty he is experiencing, his breathlessness and ankle-swelling for example, is not a normal concomitant of old age but is the consequence of a disease which requires investigation and treatment. In some cases, however, the reason that the person does not refer his problem is not that he is ignorant but that he prefers not to refer the problem. There are a number of possible reasons for such behaviour: the old person may:
1. be anxious that he will be put in an institution if he reveals that he is in difficulty
2. prefer to put up with, or 'live with', his difficulty rather than run the risk that his hopes will be raised and then dashed
3. prefer to put up with his problem rather than run the risk that he will be unable to solve it and experience feelings of inadequacy and failure
4. be reluctant to expose himself to detailed questioning about his financial situation
5. be afraid that local people will be involved as volunteers and find out personal information about him.

Many elderly people therefore maintain that they are 'all right' even when it is obvious to other people that they are in difficulty, because they prefer this course of action to admitting that they need help. Some are fully aware of the reason that they are refusing offers of help; others are completely unaware of their motives, but all adopt the same position when approached by a case-finder. This raises an ethical dilemma for the case-finder. Should he challenge the old person's statement and attempt to change her decision or accept it and leave her alone? Such a dilemma can be avoided. The more trusted the case-finder, the more likely is it that the old person will admit her problems to him, and this means that, in general, the professional who has a long-standing relationship with the old person is more likely to be told of an old person's problems than a stranger who has never met the old person before. The general practitioner is, therefore, in a good position to practise case-finding, and those who work in the same team, for example the health visitor and the district nurse in the United Kingdom, are also in a good position to discover unreported problems. If professionals with this type of relationship are prepared to visit an old person more than once, because the admission of a problem may only be made on the second or third visit, and are clear in their explanation to the old person that the objective of the exercise is to keep the old person in her own home, if that is what she wants, most problems will be revealed. However, even a well-trusted doctor may not be told of an old person's problems if the old person has adopted the attitude of 'I'm all right' as a means of coping with her problem and he will therefore have to decide how strongly to challenge the old person's point of view.

It is impossible to give general guidelines which will be useful in every case except to state the views of old people are more often challenged too weakly than too strongly. This does not mean that the views of old people should be overridden if they do not agree. In the end the old person's view that she is 'all right' may be unchanged and should be respected, but old people, like people of all ages, have a right to have their views cogently challenged. It is not a token of respect simply to accept the view of an old person with which one disagrees; it is for more respectful to argue with her, even if that causes her some distress. Argument is the stuff of human interaction, and old people have no less need of it than younger people.

EFFECTIVENESS

The effectiveness of screening is 'not proven' but case-finding, in contrast, appears to need little justification. It is obviously beneficial to elderly people who have problems which they have been unable to bring to the attention of health and social services to have such problems recognised and tackled (Lowther et al, 1970). Furthermore, case-finding can be argued to be particularly important in old age because the loss of organ reserve that characterises old age means that the effects of disabling disease are more difficult to reverse the longer the disease is left untreated.

However, case-finding has not yet been shown to be effective in preventing either the admission of old people to long-stay care or in slowing down the rate of physical deterioration. The only randomised controlled clinical trial of case-finding, conducted in Oxfordshire, England, found that it made 'no significant impact on the prevalence of medical, functional and social problems. The group receiving case finding did, however, make more use of health and social services.' (Tulloch & Moore, 1979). Research based on the Woodside Health Centre in Glasgow demonstrated that there were fewer unmet social needs and symptoms requiring intervention eight months after an initial case-finding assessment. The study measured the services which had been provided for the elderly people who had had unmet needs or symptoms identified at the initial assessment. This project certainly demonstrated that some of the unmet social needs and previously undetected symptoms were alleviated as a result of the case-finding exercise, but there was no measure of the impact of case-finding on functional ability or the burden being borne by families (Barber & Wallis, 1978).

The great majority of elderly people welcome case-finding. They find it reassuring if no serious disease is found and are encouraged that an interest is being taken in their problems. Even if their problem is insoluble or if there are insufficient resources to provide the help they need, the experience of case-finding for the old person is, in most cases, positive. It improves their quality of life and encourages a more positive attitude towards their health, which may result in a change in lifestyle or improved compliance, and which may encourage earlier self-referral should new problems develop.

Case-finding is also useful to those who plan and manage health services. The fear that the discovery of large amounts of unmet need will lead to the services being overwhelmed have proved unfounded. The discovery of unmet need does present problems to the health services, it is true. It makes the allocation of resources even more difficult, but it leads to a more effective use of resources. The greater the number of cases known to those who have to make decisions about resource allocation, the more appropriate will be the use of those resources. Case-finding therefore improves the management of resources, even though it makes life more difficult for the professional who has to manage them. Case-finding and the discovery of unmet need also improves health service planning because it allows the planner a more complete picture of the pattern of need.

Case-finding, therefore confers some benefits on elderly people, but it is difficult to distinguish the effects of the case-finding *per se* from the effect of the coincidental interventions, such as the increased number of social contacts and the warm and sympathetic interest shown by the case-finders. As a consequence of this it is inappropriate to classify those benefits as the outcome of case-finding or to assess the effectiveness of the case-finding with respect to these benefits, for they may be due to factors other than the identification of unreported problems. It is more appropriate to talk of the impact of case-finding on health in old age, and it can be stated that case-finding has a positive impact. However, the demonstration that a service has a positive impact does not justify the investment of resources. The benefits have to outweigh the benefits for elderly people that could be obtained by investing the same amount of resources in other services.

Screening and case-finding have, however, benefits other than those enjoyed by the elderly person:
1. Helping doctors to build a picture of 'normal' ageing
2. Providing more relaxed opportunities than episodes of illness to improve communication with elderly patients and their families
3. Offering opportunities to influence the knowledge and expectations of patients and their relatives about preventive and anticipatory care
4. Providing more effective health care through a planned use of resources
5. Generating pressure for additional resources through the detection and quantification of problems.

The main benefit from screening may be the reassurance many old people feel after a medical examination has failed to reveal any disease. Ferguson Anderson and Nairn Cowan emphasised this point in their description of a consultative health centre; 'It has been a delight to meet so many interesting and charming old people who have by their gratitude confirmed the belief that reassurance based on a complete physical examination is of the greatest value in maintaining morale and wellbeing' (Anderson & Cowan, 1955), while Tulloch and Moore stated that 'We formed the firm impression during the study, although there is no objective evidence to support this view, that patient morale and self-esteem would improve simply as a result of receiving special attention which several of them contrasted with the indifference society normally shows them.'

COST-EFFECTIVENESS

Screening and case-finding therefore have some benefits, but they also have costs. The application of screening tests such as those cited in Table 5.1 exposes the elderly person to an increased risk of the most common preventable disease in old age — iatrogenic disease. For example, the costs and benefits of screening for high blood pressure in old age are more difficult to calculate than the costs and benefits of screening younger people, because the beneficial effects are less and the costs, notably the incidence of drug side-effects, higher.

Another cost is the cost of resources used in screening. These can be measured in financial terms, but it is better to assess the opportunity costs, namely the cost in terms of what else could have been done with the resources used for screening. Barber and Wallis have calculated the financial cost of screening in a careful series of studies and they have argued that it is not unreasonably expensive. Barber has estimated that to set up a full screening assessment programme for over 75-year-olds (about 200) in a practice of 4000 patients would require 18 hours of health visitor (registered nurse with additional training in prevention and health education) time per week for the first year and 11 hours per week for subsequent years (Barber & Wallis, 1980a). In an attempt to reduce this time commitment, Barber has tested a postal screening questionnaire but found that about 80 per cent of his respondents still required to be seen for assessment (Barber et al, 1980). They do not, however, provide sufficient data about the level of provision of services for their population to allow the opportunity costs to be calculated, but a full costing of screening and case-finding in old age should take into account the alternative means of spending these resources — the opportunity costs. Would it, for example, have had a greater impact if those resources had been spent on the development of a weekend home nursing service or the provision of telephones or the support of the voluntary sector?

Another commonly employed strategy in preventive medicine that might reduce costs is the identification of risk factors for the purpose of selective screening. 'Risk' is a popular, but inconsistently used, term in clinical work and literature and, while it implies something about outcome, like 'prevention' itself, it is often difficult to know whether it is being used with respect to illness, accident, institutionalisation or death.

It is useful to divide risk factors into two main groups: those such as age, marital status, recent hospitalisation etc. which can be known without seeing the elderly person and which have implications for primary care record systems, and those such as mobility, mental impairment, etc. which require contact with the individual for their detection.

There are a number of attributes that are widely accepted as increasing the likelihood of functional decline and thus hospitalisation or institutionalisation. Some examples are:
1. Living alone
2. Poverty
3. Recent bereavement
4. Recent hospitalisation
5. Locomotor difficulties
6. Mental impairment.

These risk factors relate to the elderly individual, but clearly the support system is relevant. To state that living alone is a high risk factor implies that available family support confers low risk. Unfortunately the very existence of family might mean that the elderly person would reach the point of hospital or institutional care at a much later (and possibly, with respect to community rehabilitation, irreversible) stage than the failing patient who lives alone.

There are few practical guidelines for doctors on how to assess support systems to predict the likely future functional status of elderly patients, because medical practice, as yet, has not been able to operationalise the extensive social science literature on support systems.

While accepting the potential validity of these attributes, we are unsure of exactly how they can be used by the individual doctor faced with an individual patient. On the one hand it is clearly important for a family doctor to pay closer attention to the housebound 84-year-old widow than to the married, mobile, 71-year-old; but, since risk factors are based on probabilities estimated from large population studies, we must still be prepared for the unexpected and be able to consider and detect hidden problems in 'low risk' individuals. The instincts of the physician who has known a person over a long period of time cannot be underestimated.

The Medical Research Council Sociology Unit in Aberdeen has just completed a study of risk profiles in the elderly (groups included were over 80 years, recently widowed, never married, living alone, socially isolated, without children, in poor economic circumstances, recently discharged form hospital, having recent change of dwelling and divorced/separated) and although significant differences were found in, among other things, health status, they concluded that such groupings were not sensitive enough for routine use in primary care (Taylor et al, 1983).

There is, however, one group in whom 'screening' has been shown to be effective, namely old people deemed to need residential care. One study of a hundred such people resulted in thirty-two being placed more appropriately than in the old people's home they had been thought to need (Brocklehurst et al, 1978). It should, however, be emphasised that the screening of these people really meant the performance of a comprehensive physical and psychological assessment by a skilled multi-disciplinary team.

IMPLICATIONS FOR SERVICE DELIVERY, EDUCATION AND RESEARCH

There is no evidence that services should be developed to search for asymptomatic disease in old age, and both professional and public education needs to emphasise this fact. However, many elderly people are worried about their health and benefit from the reassurance that can be given following a clinical review. Such a review should include a physical examination, because the close contact that occurs during an examination is very important for some elderly people, and because signs of disease which have not been noticed or mentioned by the elderly person may be detected. It is, however, important for the doctor to consider carefully the tests he wishes to carry out in his physical examination and to be careful that his enthusiasm does not lead him to perform tests that will lead to unnecessary treatment and iatrogenic disease. For example, the doctor should only reach for the sphygmomanometer if he is confident that he knows what he will regard as 'high' when he measures the pressure and that benefits of treatment in his particular patient will outweigh the costs (Kellogg, 1983).

The problems of screening indicate the need for further research. There is, firstly, a need for more longitudinal studies which can illuminate the natural history of ageing and disease in old age. Secondly, there is a need for studies designed to assess the effectiveness of specific tests such as the measurement of high blood pressure, and there is, thirdly, a need to seek more information about the beliefs and attitudes of old people themselves. At present many old people are enthusiastic about period health examinations, but their attitudes might change if they appreciated how ineffective the search for asymptomatic disease in old age actually is.

We believe that many elderly individuals would like to have a regular, usually an annual, 'check up' mainly to confirm that they are well, with the added benefit that it maintains their relationship with 'their' personal physician. They, however, may not expect or even want a structured assessment, and in developing anticipatory and preventive strategies in our practices to help elderly patients with hidden needs we have to be aware of some unhelpful outcomes in addition to the unnecessary medical interventions mentioned above. By asking questions we may unwittingly concentrate on problems and thus reinforce the negative stereotype of ageing and reduce morale. Any medical intervention in the elderly poses the risk of 'medicalising' old age, and it may be that *what* we do is not as important as *how* we do it. Two recent randomised controlled trails demonstrate that regular visiting has a beneficial effect on elderly people (Hendricksen et al, 1984, Vetter et al, 1984) and it may well be that it is not so much the identification and solution of unreported problems that is of benefit as the development of a continuing and sustaining relationship.

REFERENCES

American College of Physicians 1981 Periodic health examinations. Annals of Internal Medicine 95: 729–732

American Medical Association 1983 Medical evaluation of healthy persons. Journal of the American Medical Association 249: 1626–1632

Anderson W F Cowan N R 1955 A consultative health centre for older people: the Rutherglen experiment. Lancet 2: 239

Barber J H, Wallis J B 1978 The benefits for an elderly population of continuing geriatric assessment. Journal of the Royal College of General Practitioners 28: 428–433

Barber J H, Wallis J B, McKeating E 1980 A postal screening questionnaire in preventive geriatric care. Journal of the Royal College of General Practitioners 30: 4951

Barber J H Wallis J B 1980a The effects of a system of geriatric screening and assessment of general practice workload. Health Bulletin 40: 125–132

Brocklehurst J C, Leeming J T, Carty M H, Robinson J M 1978 Medical screening of old people accepted for residential care. Lancet 2: 141–142

Canadian Ministry of National Health and Welfare 1979 The periodic health examination. Report of a Task Force to Conference of Deputy Ministry of Health

Charap M H 1981 The periodic health examination: genesis of a myth. Annals of Internal Medicine 95: 733–735

Cohen, Lord (of Birkenhead), Williams E T, McLachlan G (eds.) 1968 Screening in medical care: reviewing the evidence. Nuffield Provincial Hospitals Trust, Oxford University Press

Commission on Chronic Illness 1957 Prevention of chronic illness. Harvard University Press, Cambridge, Mass.

Fielding J E 1979 Prevention services for the well population. In Healthy People — the Surgeon General's Report on Health Promotion and Disease Prevention — Background Papers. US Department of Health Education and Welfare (phs) 79 - 55071A. Government Printing Office, 277–304

Hogarth J 1978 Health terminology. World Health Organisation

Hendriksen C, Lund E, Strømgärd E 1984 Consequences of assessment and intervention among elderly people. British Medical Journal 289: 1522–1524

Kellogg International Scholarship Program on Health and Aging 1983 The contribution of the primary care doctor to the medical care of the elderly in the community. Institute of Gerontology, University of Michigan, and Institute of Social Medicine, University of Copenhagen

Lowther C P, MacLeod R D M, Williamson J 1970 Evaluation of early diagnostic services for the elderly. British Medical Journal 3: 275–277

Taylor R, Ford G, Barber J H 1983 The elderly at risk. Age Concern

Tulloch A J, Moore V 1979 A randomised controlled trial of geriatric screening and surveillance in general practice. Journal of the Royal College of General Practitioners 29: 730–733

Vetter N J, Jones D A, Victor C R 1984 Effect of health visitors working with elderly patients in general practice. British Medical Journal 1: 369–372

Williamson J, Stokoe I H, Gray S, Fisher M, Smith A McGhee A, Stephenson E 1964 Old people at home: their unreported needs. Lancet 1: 1116–1120

Wilson J M G, Jungner G 1968 Principles and practice of screening for disease. Public Health Paper Number 4, WHO, Geneva

5   J. D. E. Knox

Prevention of iatrogenic disease

FROM CURE TO CARE

While this chapter has doctor activities as its main focus, it is also concerned with wider issues, such as self-care and helping those who look after the elderly (carers). General interest appears to be increasing in these aspects of care which hitherto have tended to be overshadowed by technological advances of curative medicine (Royal College of General Practitioners, 1981). This shift in emphasis is true of all age groups, and especially so in regard to those aged 65 and over. One possible reason for this change is the fact that there are more old people, and they are living longer. The figures in Table 5.1 relate to the city of Dundee, but they reflect what appears to be happening nationally in the United Kingdom.

Such increases in proportions of the old and especially the very old bring with them many problems which can and do involve doctors, especially those doctors whose job it is to provide first-contact, personal, on-going care to individuals and their families in a general practice setting.

It is widely recognised that 'old age never comes singly'. Inherent in ageing are degenerative diseases, neoplasms, metabolic and endocrine disorders

Table 5.1 The elderly population, Dundee district

	(a) Total population*	Number aged 65 and over	(%)	(b) Mean percentage of patients of 65 years and over in combined NHS lists participating doctors**
1971	197 370	25 145	(12.7)	12.2
1976	194 420	27 601	(14.2)	13.8
1979	190 793	28 185	(14.8)	14.2

Sources: *1971 Census and Tayside Regional Council
 **Tayside Area Health Board

such as Addisonian pernicious anaemia, hypothyroidism, and maturity onset diabetes. These conditions, of course, do not exist in a vacuum. It is the elderly who may also experience social isolation often associated with bereavement, 'the empty nest', retirement, rehousing, and diminished income: often such problems increase the complexities of the more purely 'medical' physical conditions.

Regular consumption of prescribed drugs may act as a crude indication of the extent to which the elderly are involved with their general practitioners. The proportion of those on regular medication rises with age, and in the very old the increase is exponential (Hall, 1981).

In the United Kingdom, social policy recognises the extra work which care of the elderly in general practice may entail, and this is reflected in additional loadings of capitation fees paid to general practitioners for the elderly on their NHS lists of patients. Having a defined list of patients confers on the British general practitioner several advantages over his counterparts in other countries: not only does the doctor have a defined denominator for any epidemiological studies he may wish to carry out, he also knows who his patients are and where they live. It is thus theoretically possible for him (and his team) to adopt a more positive and active approach to many problems which in the past have remained hidden until a crisis evokes a 'fire-brigade' response. In recent years those responsible for organising primary care service in several NHS regions have prepared lists of patients on computer file. An up-to-date practice register is thus readily available to NHS general practitioners in these regions.

Opportunities for special efforts for the elderly in a practice population must be viewed against a background of needs, demands and expectations.

Williamson et al (1964) were among the first to record the unmet needs of the elderly surveyed in the setting of general practice. Reasons for these unmet needs included low expectations held at that time by many of the elderly in relation to both their ideas of health and to what health services might have to offer them. Personal experience leads the author to suspect that the scene is changing: older people, now more aware of social policy and of their own situations, tend to make increasing demands on their general practitioner. As one old-age pensioner put it, 'He [the doctor] gets paid to visit once every month, so why doesn't he?' Of course this is a misinterpretation of the NHS system of payment, but it illustrates the point.

Expectations must be taken into consideration by planners in attempts to balance the (so far) insoluble equation of matching needs to demands, and both to limited resources. In addition, any account written from the standpoint of the general practitioner must include the whole context in which general practice care is provided. This is because, at the level of the individual patient, it is the general practitioner who decides what priorities to allot the many different elements in the day-to-day work of the practice.

Primary medical care — current practice

Unlike most other specialties, general practice is not a uniform entity: its context, practice organisation and practice policies differ — sometimes very markedly — from one geographical area to another. Many determinants influence the degree of priority which general practitioners accord to the care of the elderly in their practices. A practice set in a young housing estate is more likely to focus on the needs of children and young mothers; because resources (including time) are finite, any shift in priorities towards greater involvement in the care of the elderly in such a practice might have to occur *at the expense of* care that practice provides for the young. The traditions of the practice, the way it has consciously (and often unconsciously) educated its patients (there is some truth in the observation that general practitioners get the patients they deserve!) and, not least, the professional interests of the doctor, are among other determinants of priorities. Accordingly, generalisations may need qualification to take account of individual exceptions: broad statements may need to be interpreted with care.

How and to what extent have general practitioners actually responded to the challenges posed by increasing proportions of elderly patients in their practices? At present there are remarkably few studies on this point. Wilson (1982) recorded virtually no change in the pattern of his work in a semi-rural practice over eighteen years. Jacob and his colleagues (1984) sampled all the work of comparable practices over a decade in Dundee: relevant findings include a small increase in the proportion of all contacts with those aged 65 years and over, a holding-steady of home visiting of the elderly against a falling overall rate, and fairly marked increase in 'indirect' consultations, over 90 per cent of which were concerned with repeat prescribing. From this evidence it appears that responses from general practice to the challenge of increasing proportions of the elderly have tended to be passive rather than active, though some notable exceptions are on record (Allibone, 1981; Hodes, 1973; Thompson, 1979).

General practitioners, like all clinicians, have a repertoire which is limited. McGregor et al (1970), in a study of effects of attaching a nursing team to a large group practice, were able to use a relatively simple classification covering the range of general practitioner activities, e.g. history, local examination, and issue of prescriptions and certificates. Other 'para-clinical' activities (such as administration and correspondence) and 'extra-practice' work (such as committees, insurance medicals, etc.) were also recorded. This study indicates clearly the interdependent nature of the work of doctors and nurses in general practice, a point which will be more fully developed later.

Prescribing occupies a central position in this repertoire. There are many reasons for this, some straightforward and obvious (for example, securing for the patient rapid freedom from symptoms), and others more complex, as will be discussed below.

DRUGS

The prescribing (and non-prescribing) of medicines is an important doctor activity, to be viewed in a wider context which should also include self-medication. Studies by Dunnell & Cartwright (1972) and others have shown that self-medication with over-the-counter drugs is more common than prescribed medication: for example, for every prescribed item taken by people in the Dunnell and Cartwright survey, there were two non-prescribed items in a two-week period. The elderly took as many over-the-counter medicines as did those under 65 years of age. The distribution by therapeutic groups of non-prescribed medicines differs from that of prescribed medication, with analgesics and medicines for the digestive system being the most common over-the-counter preparations. There is evidence that, like prescribed medication, self-medication is uncreasing. In addition, there is the possibility that elderly patients may hoard prescribed medicines which they may take later without medical supervision. Personal experience has shown that where elderly people are grouped together (as in 'enclaves' of sheltered housing), a certain amount of swapping of drugs goes on. Most of this relates to less potent drugs, and serves a variety of needs, possibly as much psychological and social as purely 'medical'. Apart from sporadic reports of adverse effects of habituation to such drugs as purgatives. there is little evidence that significant harm results from self-medication. It may, however, increase the risk of interactions with prescribed drugs. How often do we as doctors make purposeful attempts to define the extent of this patient activity before we prescribe? Might there be scope for attempting to modify such self-medication by health visitors and doctors?.

Prescribed medicines

Studies such as those by Law & Chalmers (1976) show that prescribing is age-related, with a steep rise in those aged 75 years and over. The content of such prescribed medication is uniform throughout the United Kingdom, with psychotropic drugs and analgesics at the top of the list, followed by diuretics, drugs acting on the cardio-vascular system, 'tonics', drugs acting on the respiratory system, and a range of others bringing up the rear.

Many of these drugs are recognised as potent therapeutic weapons. When confronted with such a list of drugs, the general practitioner can usually justify his actions in prescribing most of them. Tulloch (1981) reviewed 175 elderly patients having regular repeat prescriptions and, in terms of prescribing costs, assessed 62 per cent of the prescriptions as 'necessary', 28 per cent as 'equivocal', and only 10 per cent as 'unnecessary'. This study did not take the patients' opinions into account, and, where potent therapeutic agents are concerned, such an emphasis on professionally assessed need at the expense of lay-conditioned demand is appropriate. Nevertheless, patients' (and relatives') wishes in relation to long-term medication cannot be ignored, as studies by Marinker and colleagues (Balint et al, 1970) have shown.

Some drugs prescribed for the elderly

Although virtually any drug may be prescribed for elderly patients, this section will be concerned with only three broad groups of medicines — first, psychotropics, second, diuretics, because they are the most commonly prescribed, while the third group comprises a miscellaneous collection, selected for their particular relevance to the theme of prevention of iatrogenic disease.

Psychotropics and analgesics

The various sleep disturbances associated with ageing (such as difficulty in falling asleep, shortened duration of sleep and frequent wakenings) are so common as to be regarded as normal. Those who week their general practitioner's help for insomnia often appear to be well aware of this fact, but the knowledge does little to help. Just as their forebears were so often preoccupied with the state of their bowels, the elderly today appear to be more concerned with insomnia. Short courses of rapidly metabolised hypnotics probably do no harm, and may give considerable relief when the main problem is difficulty in falling asleep. However, tolerance is rapidly acquired, and both patient and doctor are tempted to increase the dose. The resultant hangover effect may be associated with an increased liability to falls. The matron of one residential home for the elderly noted a sharp decrease in the entries in the 'accident book' coincidental with a reduction in frequency and dose of hypnotics among the residents.

At the time of writing, the author's conscious preference when faced with the need to prescribe for the elderly is for temazepam (Euhypnos) or triazolam (Halcion). Yet a recent analysis of his prescribing, while confirming the high proportion of hypnotics in the psychotropic group, revealed that in fact nitrazepam, often in the relatively high does of 10 mg at night, was the commonest prescribed hypnotic. This difference between observed and expected findings illustrates the need for some kind of prescribing audit, which is discussed later.

Confusion is another relatively frequently encountered phenomenon, usually a later manifestation of senile dementia. Drug therapy is unlikely to improve this condition, which may in fact be induced by many different medications, e.g. hypnotics, anti-depressants, digoxin. This is a further factor to be taken into account before prescribing any medication in the elderly.

Generalised muscle stiffness, aches and pains, are among other frequent complaints. Such locomotor symptomatology is commonly associated with degenerative joint disease. Proprietary non-striodal anti-inflammatory agents have been aggressively promoted; while they may afford considerable relief, nevertheless it appears that in general the therapeutic ratio of such drugs is reduced in the elderly. Indomethacin and related drugs may precipitate congestive failure because of associated fluid retention, and, in the author's practice, during the past five years at least three elderly patients have had significant gastro-intestinal haemorrhages necessitating hospital admission which were associated with NSAID therapy. The Opren, Zomax and more recent Osmosin stories are further illustrations of the need for increased caution in relation to newly introduced analgesics. There is still a place for dispersable aspirin to be taken with food, or paracetamol in regular and adequate doses.

Diuretics

One of the 'quiet revolutions' of therapeuticvs for the elderly occurring within the author's professional lifetime has been the emergence of oral diuretics as drug treatment of first choice in lesser degress of congestive failure. This therapy has become the key to long-term management of leg oedema of many other types — including ankle swelling from the enforced immobility of the aged, varicose veins, and 'idiopathic oedema'. The impact this revolution has had on domiciliary nursing practice has not received due recognition; no longer are nurses (and patients) tied to a relatively inflexible regime of twice-weekly 'mersalyl' by injection. The patient and doctor now have greater freedom to tune treatment more nicely to suit the condition, while nurse has been freed to devote more of her time to essentially nursing procedures. It is little wonder that general practitioners have welcomed this development, and sometimes may be seen to prescribe oral diuretics perhaps too readily. In theory, the risks are moderately great, with possibilities of precipitating electrolyte (especially potassium) depletion, gout and diabetes mellitus. A recent monitoring exercise in the author's own practice, however, revealed no evidence of major problems, despite a policy of reserving potassium supplements only for those patients undergoing purposeful therapy to shift significant oedema, while allowing those on maintenance therapy to obtain added potassium from natural food sources such as fresh oranges. Nevertheless, it may still be useful to ensure as far as possible that each old person on maintenance diuretic therapy should have at least a yearly biochemical check on urea and electrolyte blood levels.

Miscellaneous drugs

Among the common and distressing complaints of the very old is dizziness, a symptom which may have several different causes; yet full investigation is relatively unrewarding because the pay-off, in terms of finding a remediable condition, is negligible. In these circumstances most general practitioners opt for drug treatment on an empirical basis. Prochlorperazine maleate (Stemetil) has achieved some popularily, probably largely as a result of commercial promotion, despite the fact that the drug can induce dizziness: it is this author's view that this drug should be used with much greater discrimination, if at all.

There are still many elderly patients who become obsessed by the behaviour (or, as they see it, misbehaviour) of their bowels. The stimulants and irritants of yesterday — cascara sagrada, castor oil and senna — have given way to bulk producers or combinations of drugs which act synergistically, e.g. Dorbanex. Such preparations appear to be better tolerated and, in the author's experience, long-term therapy has not led to the spastic constipation formerly seen in association with habituation to irritant purgatives.

The harm we may do

Prescribing, particularly in relation to the elderly, is usually a matter of swings and roundabouts — therapeutic goals to be achieved at some cost, to be measured in various ways, including risks to the patient's wellbeing: physical, psychological and social.

One of the reasons for including this chapter is the greatly increased potential for unintended harm to our patients inherent in prescribing for the elderly. The reasons for this potential for harm are numerous. In relation to the prescribed medicines themselves, increased potency often resides in a narrowed 'therapeutic ratio' of effectiveness to adverse effect. In the elderly the pharmacokinetics of drugs with the slowing of metabolic processes may enhance the possibility of adverse reactions.

Old age is often associated with increasing forgetfulness and confusion, leading to increased risk of over-and under-dosing. Diseases are often age-related: several different diseases may often coexist, leading to an increased potential for drug interactions. It has been shown that, on average, old people are prescribed about three times as many medicines as those aged under 65 years.

Numerous examples of avoidable harm have been recorded, including adverse reactions (such as skin eruption), undue toxicity from inadvertent overdosing, toxicity from undue sensitivity and from interactions of incompatible drugs.

In addition to such physical effects, there is the possibility of enhancing a dependence on doctors inherent in each act of prescribing. Here is an example: To help Mrs A cope with the transient sleep disturbance associated with the death of her husband, she was given a small supply of nitrazepam 5 mag. Six years later she still attends at intervals determined by the supply of her tablets, which she continues to request and the doctor continues to supply, possibly because doctor and patient feel a need to 'legitimise' these contacts by focussing on hypnotic drugs.

While the potential for harm is considerable, the reality is, fortunately, not as serious as has been feared. Over-emphasis on the problem stems from an uncritical extrapolation into the general community of studies which in fact are narrowly based on subsections of the population admitted to hospital. In addition, at least one study in general practice gave unduly adverse results, based on a number of misinterpretations of the data. Poor compliance may not necessarily harm the patient — it has even been suggested that it may exert a protective effect!

Towards safer prescribing

Before reaching for his prescription pad, the doctor faced by an elderly patient needs to consider such issues as the following:
1. What alternatives, if any, are there to prescribing for this patient?
2. Am I prescribing the drug purely for pharmacological therapeutic reason; if not, what other reasons might there be?
3. Is the patient sufficiently responsible to cope with a pharmacological approach to management?
4. Do I know enough about the drug I am about to prescribe to be in a position to calculate possible risks?
5. What other medicines (prescribed and over-the-counter) might this patient be taking?
6. If any other drugs are being administered, is significant harm likely to accrue if I stop at least one of them before introducing another?
7. How soon can I discontinue this drug?

Towards better compliance

Although Drury et al (1976) have shown that compliance in general practice is significantly better than among patients supervised by hospital clinics, there is room for improvement in regard to the elderly.

Atkinson and colleagues (1978) include the following elements in a list of ways of improving compliance:
1. Ensuring the patient understands what is required by the proposed regime, e.g. giving the elderly in hospital a chance to be responsible for their own drug regime *before* discharge home
2. minimising possible confusion by adhering to one paricular brand of tablet
3. Taking into account any views the patient may have about the taste, colour and other aspects of the proposed medication
4. Providing contains with screw caps which are easily removed (and are clearly labelled).

Largely for economic reasons the Health Departments wish to encourage the widespread adoption of generic prescribing within the next few years in the United Kingdom. Wade (1983), writing from experience in his practice, has recorded problems encountered by patients who have found alternative forms of their particular medicine to be less effective. He also draws attention to the removal of the patient's visual check on their own medication which blanket introduction of generic prescribing might entail. He advocates the introduction of an acceptable identification code *before* generic prescribing is widely adopted, to minimise possible confusion in patients' minds.

To ensure the elderly clearly understand their drugs and doses, some doctors provide a card with sample tablets/capsules affixed by transparent adhesive tape, and opposite each formulation a note of the name of the drug, what it is supposed to do, and the frequency with which it should be taken.

Some doctors advocate the use of special pre-packed containers which will automatically dispense the medicines day by day. A simpler approach to this problem is to use seven of the spaces for eggs in a twelve-egg container, each of which may be painted a different colour for a day of the week. Each week the container is prepacked by the patient, or by a relative if responsibility for medication is in doubt.

The problem of ensuring the correct dose of the appropriate drug to the right person at the right time is much more complex in residential homes for the elderly. Knox & Melvin (1980) have described the use of individualised containers in trays in an attempt to minimise possible errors and improve compliance in such circumstances.

Most general practitioners share their chronic visiting list with other members of the primary health care team — nursing sister and health visitor. All concerned with the on-going professional supervision of a patient on long-term medication can collaborate (and communicate) in monitoring compliance.

Towards safer repeat prescribing

Maintaining supplies of drugs without seeing the patient on each reissue of a prescription has become increasingly prevalent. Provided this repeat prescribing is operated under some system, possible dangers to the patient are minimal. Essential elements of a system include:
1. Providing the patient with a card on which are listed details concerning all long-term drugs, together with spaces for dates and drugs (usually coded by number) actually issued
2. Providing in the general practitioner medical record a similar chart, together with reasons for long-term medication and dates when the patient should be seen and prescribing reviewed.

The receptionist often acts as the key operator of the system, and writes out the prescription. This should of course be checked and signed by the doctor. Such prescriptions may be posted to the patient or held in a secure place at reception for personal handing over to the patient or the patient's recognised representative. Such systems, reviewed by Drury (1973), usually work well and help maintain standards of individual patient care. They do not give a general picture of the practice prescribing habits, however. This overview can be obtained by analysis of carbon copies of prescriptions sampled over a period. Health authorities can also make available to the prescribing NHS general practitioner all his or her prescriptions in a sample month, after the scripts have been processed by the Pricing Authority. By the time such prescriptions become available, however, many months have passed, and the doctor may have difficulty relating individual prescriptions to particular patients and remembering the circumstances surrounding the issue of the prescription.

Recently, methods of providing both the individual repeat prescription and a record of all such prescriptions have been developed using the microcomputer and line printer (Meldrum, 1982). This information is a prerequisite for any form of audit, and is greatly facilitated by a computer.

Groups of doctors, usually working in health centres, are also beginning to develop, by mutual agreement, their own practice formularies in attempts to improve their prescribing and to introduce systems of self-audit (Table 5.2).

Alternatives to prescribing

Although prescribing occupies, or appears to occupy, a central place in doctor activities, it is only part of therapeutic activity which in a broader sense is a component of patient management. For example: Mrs B was given increasing doses of temazepam in unsuccessful attempts to control the nocturnal excursions associated with her senile dementia. However, when Mrs B's attendances at day hospital were increased from once to four times weekly, her insomnia became more manageable. The fatigue engendered in Mrs B allowed the dose of temazepam to be reduced, to the benefit of herself and her family.

Thus, by increasing other components of management, it may become possible to decrease prescribing of psychotropic drugs. The availability and accessibility of a doctor who knows his or her patient are possibly significant in this context, because out-of-hours visits made by doctors working in

Table 5.2 Auditing prescribing

Suggested goals

The undermentioned suggestions might provide useful points for debate in a practice meeting relating to prescribing:

1. *Patients on maintenance oral diuretic therapy*
    a. At what intervals would you agree the serum potassium level should be assessed?
    b. Should the urine be tested for sugar? If so, at what intervals of time?

2. *Patients on maintenance B_{12}*
    How frequently should the haemoglobin be estimated?

3. *Patients on long-term psychotropics*
    How frequently should the need/demand for these be discussed with the patient?

4. *Patients on long-term digoxin*
    Which patients in your practice who are receiving digoxin might be considered for discontinuing the drug?

deputising services are thought to be associated with increased likelihood of admission to hospital and prescribing. Home visiting is another item of management which the following 'cameo' suggests may play a part: Mrs C told her son to inform her general practitioner that, in place of the prescription for another drug he had sent in response to her telephone call, she would have preferred another visit.

Each general practitioner has a visiting list of 'chronics' and the elderly; some of these visits may be shared with nursing staff and health visitors. Such collaboration needs the backing of community nursing administrators and teamwork within the practice staff.

Allibone (1981) claims that most communities have a great untapped resource in volunteers with potential skills to assist in overcoming the social isolation of the elderly. He mobilised more than 200 volunteers in his community, and found that their work 'has immeasurably improved social contact of the isolated elderly people in our villages'. His report makes no mention of possible effects of such contact on his prescribing however.

There is evidence that some confused elderly patients can be reorientated for time and place using the technique of 'reality orientation'. While most of the relevant work so far carried out relates to patients in institutions, there may be a place for applying the techniques to patients in the community. Demented elderly living with relatives and attending geriatric day hospitals would be in a position to receive 'reality orientation' therapy in a consistent and systematic way. Results of one empirical study of this approach to the confused elderly at home suggest that the improvement observed at day hospital was matched by changes in the patients' behaviour at home, and an easing of the stress on relatives (Greene et al, 1983).

TEAM AND TEAMWORK

Current views on the primary health care team in the United Kingdom focus particularly on the general practitioner, together with his or her receptionist staff, nursing sister and health visitor (Department of Health and Social Security, 1981). By frequent contact, each may come to recognise the professional contributions others make to patients and the community. The exchange of information at such contacts can promote the delivery of more efficient and effective care than is otherwise possible. At such meetings the doctor can update his or her knowledge of the patients' circumstances and often plan future developments in providing care in a coordinated manner. This sharing of care is unlikely to happen by itself if too strict a view is held of confidentiality or if the attitude of any of the professionals involved is too authoritarian. In addition, there are potential management problems in marrying a hierarchical system of administration (characteristic of nursing) with the greater egalitarianism of general practice. For these and other reasons, teamwork among the core staff in general practice is still relatively unchanged.

It is possible to take a wider view of who constitutes the team, to include social workers. Where management of the elderly (and the inherent potential to modify prescribing) so often involves action to alleviate loneliness, to reinforce the day-to-day care by relatives, and to ensure appropriate housing, it makes sense for general practitioners and social workers to collaborate. Yet examples of such collaboration are still the exception rather than the rule.

The retail pharmacist is another professional who, viewed from general practice, is often seen to be somewhat peripheral. However, his contribution to the prevention of iatrogenic disease is important: he may prompt the prescribing doctor to amend errors in prescriptions, and he may provide the elderly with helpful advice on health problems and on the use of primary care services. His potential special role in operating a safer system of prescribed medicines in residential homes for the elderly has been described by Knox & Melvin (1980).

Collaboration with hospital

It is well known that the advantages of admission of the elderly to hospital are offset by a number of disadvantages, such as the precipitation of an episode of confusion, and an additional mortality risk. The concept of centralisation of hospital services at the expense of 'community hospitals' may increase the social isolation of the elderly. The longer duration of stay and slower turnover of bed associated with the elderly has considerable implications for the acute sector of hospital services, and for undergraduate medical education, still based virtually entirely on hospitals. Not least among disadvantages is the cost of the inappropriately placed elderly patient whose main needs are often nursing rather than technological care.

Such arguments potentiate the wish of the elderly themselves to continue to be cared for at home during periods of illness. It is sometimes possible to increase temporarily the level of nursing and other care to meet such needs and, at the time of writing, this 'home hospital' concept is being evaluated.

On a less acute level, collaboration between general practitioners and geriatricians can extend to include anticipatory care. On recognising an elderly patient likely to run into trouble in the foreseeable future, the family doctor initiates action to acquaint the geriatric services with the situation at a stage where little or no action is required. Should transfer to institutional care be needed later, admission is thereby facilitated. This system of anticipatory care includes provision of periodic short spells of respite for caring relatives of the elderly. Well in advance of statutory holidays, short-term residential care — in a 'home', or hospital, if need be — is planned to free the relative for a much-needed break. This form of support, in the author's experience, has allowed frail elderly people to continue to be cared for in their own surroundings; in the absence of such a system, much avoidable morbidity may be induced in the carers and early breakdown of support at home will result in avoidable institutionalisation of the elderly — both, in a sense, iatrogenic phenomena.

One of the ill effects of current adverse economic circumstances is the threat of cutting back social services, including home helps. As a result, the ability to maintain an elderly patient at home is threatened, and the general practitioner may be forced to seek hospital admission, with the potential for iatrogenic disease, for a patient whose problems are more social than medical. Action to prevent such an eventuality is political rather than medical, and is more difficult because it is not likely to attract votes in an election.

ACCORDING PRIORITIES

More needs to be done to meet the needs of a growing section of the community, and one especially at risk to iatrogenic disease, especially from prescribed medicines. Altering prescribing is not simply a matter of telling general practitioners to curb this activity. Additional time has to be found, time to listen, time to visit, time to compile a practice register, time to find out to what extent the needs of the elderly are known and are being met.

The action to be taken will usually require coordinated teamwork, and this calls for changes in priorities and in training of the health professionals. The general practitioner could be offered an additional incentive: possibly the amount saved by more efficient and economic prescribing could be made available to the practice to employ a nursing sister devoted entirely to monitoring the elderly.

Health authorities, and posssibly the discipline of community medicine, could collaborate by providing *all* general practitioners with computerised lists of the over-65s in their practices, and by epidemiological studies based on such lists. The community medicine specialist could provide a resource needed to make audit of prescribing and of quality of medical care of the elderly a more routine activity. Society itself needs to be made more aware of the potential hazards of 'a pill for every ill' type of philosophy. Health education endeavours to highlight the risks of prescribed medication in pregnancy have been remarkably successful: perhaps similar efforts could be made on behalf of the elderly.

REFERENCES

Allibone A 1981 It does work. British Medical Journal 283: 1581–1582
Atkinson L, Gibson I, Andrews J 1978 An investigation into the ability of elderly patients continuing to take drugs after dischange from hospital and recommendations concerning improving the situation. Gerontology 24: 225–234
Balint M, Hunt J, Joyce D, Marinker M, Woodcock J 1970 Treatment or Diagnosis. A study of repeat prescriptions in general practice. Tavistock, London
Drury V W M 1973 Repeat prescription cards. Journal of the Royal College of General Practitioners 23: 511–514
Drury V W M, Wade O L, Woolf E 1976 Following advice in general practice. Journal of the Royal College General Practitioners 26: 712–718
Dunnell K, Cartwright A 1972 Medicine Takers, Prescribers and Hoarders. Routledge and Kegan Paul, London.

Greene J G, Timbury G C, Smith R, Gardiner M 1983 Reality orientation with elderly patients in the community: an empirical evaluation. Age and Ageing 12: 38–43
Hall M S 1981 Prescribing frequency and costs related to patients' age and sex Practitioner 225: 271–273
Hodes C 1973 Care of the elderly in general practice. British Medical Journal 4: 41–42
Knox J D E, Anderson R A, Jacob A, Campion P D 1984 general practitioners' care of the elderly: studies of aspects of workload. Journal of the Royal College of General Practitioners 34: 194–198
Knox J D E, Melvin M 1980 Prescribed medicines in a residential home for the elderly. Nursing Times 1934–1936
Law R, Chalmers C 1976 Medicines and elderly people: a general practice survey. British Meidical Journal 1: 565–568
McGregor S W, Heasman M A, Kuenssberg E V 1971 The evaluation of a direct nursing attachment in a north Edinburgh practice. Scottish Health Service Studies No 18, Scottish Home and Health Department.
Meldrum D 1982 Computerized repeat prescription control. Update 24: 2167–2175
Murdoch J C 1980 The epidemiology of prescribing in an urban general practice. Journal of the Royal College of General Practitioners 30: 593–602
The Primary Health Care Team 1981 Report of a Joint Working Group of the Standing Medical Advisory Committee and the Standing Nursing and Midwifery Advisory Committee, Department of Health and Social Security
Royal College of General Practitioners 1981 Health and Prevention in Primary Care. Report from General Practice No 18, Royal College of General Practitioners
Thompson M K 1979 The care of the older patient in winter. Practitioner 223: 787-791
Tulloch A J 1981 Practice research: repeat prescribing for elderly patients. British Medical Journal 282: 1672–1675
Wade A G 1983 Generic prescribing. British Medical Journal 287: 985
Williamson J, Stokoe I H, Gray S, Fisher M, Smitth A, McGhee A, Stephenson E 1964 Old people at home: their unreported needs. Lancet: 1:1117–1120
Wilson J B 1982 Workload in a rural practice over the past eighteen years. Lancet 1: 733–734

6   *J. A. Muir Gray, E. J. Bassey and A. Young*

The risks of inactivity

INTRODUCTION

The opening chapter of this book emphasised how little is known about the natural history of ageing. Cross-sectional studies offer only limited insights because they provide no data about the experience of each cohort as it ages. and even longitudinal studies have their limitations because the longitudinal study of one cohort does not allow the effect of secular trends to be discerned unless a series of cohorts are followed. Valid population studies are therefore difficult and expensive. It is, however, possible to obtain some ideas about the natural history of ageing by considering a hypothetical individual and trying to consider the reasons for the changes that take place in that individual as he grows older. Let us consider one change — the progressive decline in his capacity for work, usually measured with respect to his maximum levels of oxygen consumption and called his maximal aerobic power, or VO_2 max (Fig. 6.1).

The capacity to work increases from birth until a peak is reached. This is usually at, or just after, the phase of physical growth and development has come to an end, namely the end of adolescence. After the maximum capacity has been reached there is usually a progressive decline, the precise age at which the decline begins varying from one individual to another, as does the rate of decline.

In few people is the rate of decline that which it would be were it due only to the normal ageing process. In most people the decline is due to both the ageing process and to a loss of fitness. A gap opens up between an individual's best posssible work capacity and his actual work capacity. This gap has been called 'the fitness gap' (Fig. 6.2).

The term 'fitness' may be used to describe an individual's maximum capacity for work. There is, however, another use of the term 'fitness' that is particularly relevant in old age, and that is that fitness may be measured not only with respect to a body's maximum capacity but also with respect to its response to a sub-maximal workload. The fitter the person, using this definition of the term, the less is the displacement of pulse, respiratory rate, and other relevant variables from their resting levels when he performs work. The

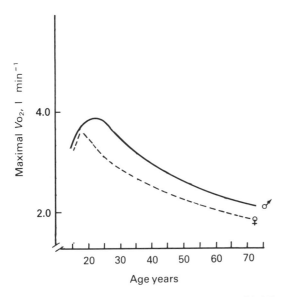

Fig. 6.1 Mean values for maximal oxygen uptake expressed in $l\ O_2\ min^{-1}$.

fitter a person, the less is his body disturbed by work and the more quickly will his body return to the resting state when the work is finished.

For the young person a loss of fitness will be significant if he is required to perform heavy work, to play rugby for example. He will however, have sufficient reserves to cope with the demands of everyday life, for example climbing stairs, walking to the pub, carrying in coal, cutting the grass, or walking to and from nearby shops. His loss of fitness will therefore neither interfere with his social life nor his ability to look after himself. If he wants to play sport, he will train to do so; if he does not, only his quality of life will be impaired by his loss of fitness. In contrast, the old person whose capacity for work is lower to start with may find that loss of fitness of the same degree will tip the balance between integration and isolation, or between independence and dependence.

It is now accepted that many of the age-related changes that were once assumed to be solely the result of the ageing process are partly the result of disuse, because they have been observed in young people confined to bed and in astronauts who have experienced prolonged periods of weightlessness (Table 6.1).

HEALTH BELIEFS AND ATTITUDES

However, disuse is not a normal concomitant of ageing. It occurs because of the prevailing beliefs and attitudes about ageing and because of disabling disease. The former have an effect on virtually all of the population, the latter only on the minority who develop such a disease.

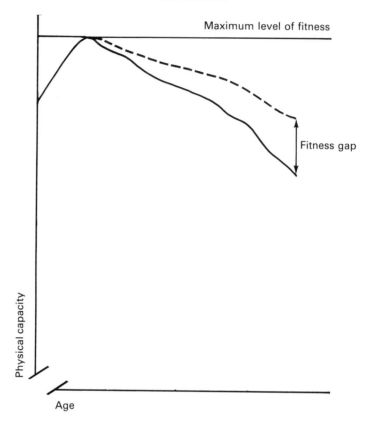

Fig. 6.2 Rate of change of physical fitness with age. Broken line is the rate of decline due to ageing alone if fitness is not lost. Continuous line is the actual rate of decline (Gray, 1982)

'Being grown-up'

The function of play has fascinated psychologists and sociologists for many years, but no single theory has emerged to explain its function. What has emerged, however, is the appreciation that it is not only children who play games

The state of being grown-up is traditionally associated with a move from play to work, but many games are played by grown-ups at work, as the social psychologists, and good novelists, have clearly demonstrated. However, the play of grown-ups differs from the play of children in many respects, one of which is of particular importance for the physical health of grown-ups, namely the decline in the amount of physical activity involved in the games adults play during the working day and in the course of family and social life. In part this is due to a loss of opportunity, but it is also due to the prevailing attitudes towards physical activity. It is not regarded as appropriate grown-up behaviour to indulge in vigorous physical activity except as part of sports

Table 6.1 Changes commonly assumed to be the result of normal ageing but which have been observed in young people or those experiencing weightlessness from Bortz W M 1982 Disuse and Aging. Journal of the American Medical Association 248: 1203–1208

Decrease in	Increase in
Vo_2 Max	Systolic blood pressure
Cardiac output	Peripheral resistance
Stroke volume	Intolerance to tilting
Plasma volume	
Lean body mass	
Bone density	
Insulin sensitivity	

or active hobbies, even though 'grown-ups' need physical activity every bit as frequently as children if they are not to lose fitness. For example, primary-school children are in no more need of regular physical activity than people in their twenties and thirties, such as their teachers, yet it is the former who are physically active during morning break and lunchtime, while the latter sit and drink coffee.

The older a person becomes the less likely he is to take physical activity of sufficient intensity, sufficiently often to maintain his level of fitness, a truism which may be called, somewhat sententiously, the law of inverse activity levels.

'Being too old for sport'

In most people a marked decline in activity levels can be observed on leaving school or university if their work does not necessitate it. Some, however, continue to remain active after leaving formal education by participating in sports or hobbies that require physical activity of the appropriate frequency, intensity and duration to maintain their level of fitness. Such people offset the harmful physical effects of grown-up inactivity by participating in a type of physical play acceptable for grown-ups, for example tennis, squash or rugby. Until recently, however, it was customary for people to indulge in such vigorous sports only while they, and their relatives and friends, considered them young enough to do so and to reach a point at which it was decided that they were 'too old' and that they should 'hang up their boots'. The precise age at which this decision was made varied from individual to individual and from sport to sport; it is customary for people to give up rugby or other contact sports before tennis, for example. There are physical reasons for such decisions, of course, but the principal reasons are social and psychological; in part the prevailing expectations and social pressures, for example getting married, lead the player to decide that he will give up; in part the social and psychological reasons that reduce the motivation of the player to win and therefore to train as he grows older. In times past it was customary for players who 'hung up their boots' to cease all physical activity, while not reducing, and sometimes increasing, their food or alcohol intake. The result was obviously a rapid loss of fitness. This is now changing, and many people are prepared to play sport to an older age. Those sports which continue to be enjoyable to most participants, whatever their age, for example cycling or tennis, have players of all ages, whereas in those sports in which participation does become more difficult, notably the contact sports, players either graduate to a less violent stratum, for example by joining a team of former first-team players who play committedly but cleanly against similar teams from other clubs, or they take up some new sport, which may be just as demanding, although less damaging.

DISABLING DISEASE

By definition, disabling diseases result in a decline in functional ability, but only a proportion of that decline is actually due to the pathological process. In almost all disease the effects resulting from the impairment caused by the diseases are compounded by the effects of disuse, both local and general. Whether the basic impairment is weakness, or stiffness, or pain, the affected individual makes less use of the affected part of the body, if one part of the body is specifically affected, and generally becomes less active, with the result that fitness is lost and the fitness gap grows even wider (Fig. 6.2).

THE IMPACT OF LOST FITNESS

A general definition of fitness was given in the introduction to his chapter; the fitter a person is, the less is his body disturbed when asked to perform additional work. The general definition, though accurate, is, necessarily, couched in vague terms. More specific terms relate to the four different aspects of physical fitness, all of which begin with the letter S — strength, stamina, skill and suppleness (Table 6.2).

Table 6.2 The four aspects of fitness

Aspect of fitness	Principal systems involved	Result of loss of fitness
Strength	Muscular	Weakness
Suppleness	Articular	Stiffness
Stamina	Cardiovascular Muscular	Breathlessness Fatigability
Skill	Central nervous	Unsteadiness Loss of ability to care for oneself

Table 6.3 British Veterans' cycling records, 1983

25 miles		50 miles		100 miles	
Age	Time	Age	Time	Age	Time
42	52.17	42	1.47.10	43	3.51.25
43	52.45	43	1.47.38	44	3.55.32
47	53.28	48	1.48.52	55	3.59.53
56	53.52	49	1.51.54	66	4.16.37
59	55.15	51	1.52.24	69	4.27.15
60	55.25	66	1.52.41	71	4.35.40
65	57.00	69	2.07.37	74	4.53.27
66	57.05	71	2.10.19	76	5.16.53
68	1.02.20	72	2.19.28		
71	1.02.53	77	2.19.57		
72	1.05.23	78	2.52.38		
73	1.06.17				
74	1.06.51				
76	1.06.53				
77	1.08.52				
81	1.23.22				
82	1.37.00				

CAN FITNESS BE MAINTAINED?

In the modern world, few types of employment prevent a loss of fitness, and of those that do strength is the only aspect of fitness that is maintained. In very few jobs outside professional sport, ballet or circus life are there sufficient demands to maintain stamina, suppleness or skills, other than those skills directly related to the job itself. Nevertheless, a small proportion of the population manage to maintain their fitness and decline at a rate determined principally by the ageing process. The actual rate of decline of such people differs little from the best possible rate of decline and the fitness gap remains small.

This group is composed of those who continue to participate in sports or who continue to have physically active hobbies throughout life, and the proportion of athletes who remain active appears to be increasing as the growing popularity of Masters Athletics Championships and Veteran Time Trials Cycling races demonstrates. The achievements of those who remain active are startling, as the records of the Veterans Times Trials Association illustrate (Table 6.3).

Conclusions drawn from studies of such people have, however, to be treated with great caution for the following reasons.
1. They are not a random sample of the population; they were, in general, fitter and had a higher capacity than the rest of the population when they were young.
2. The sample itself is continually modified by the loss of those who die or who become disabled.
3. Athletes have lower prevalence of cigarette smoking than those who are not athletes.

Table 6.4 Secular trends in U.K Veterans Cycling Records

Event	Age of record holder	1972	1982
25 mile solo	56	58.39	53.52
	65	1. 3.39	57.00
	76	1.15.55	1.06.53
100 mile solo	55	3.59.53*	4.23.12
	66	4.41.31	4.16.37
	76	5.17.12	5.16.53
12 hours	55	241.2 miles	260.5 miles
	66	228.6 miles	243.3 miles
	75	207.5 miles	207.5 miles**

* No 1972 record for 55-year-old: record for 53-year-old cyclist given
** Record set in 1970 by H.A. Wenman
Note: Ages in the table were selected to be as close as possible to 55, 65 and 75; comparable data for these ages is not available.

4. The prevalence of obesity is lower among athletes.
5. 'Elderly athletes' are not a homogenous group and one cohort of elderly athletes differs from another.
6. Secular trends also cause difficulties in interpretation. The records of older athletes are improving, as Table 6.4 demonstrates, but the decreasing weight of bikes and the progressive improvement in road surfaces and increasing competitiveness of elderly athletes may all be relevant.

In a review of the evidence about the ageing athlete, Shephard cautiously concluded that 'both longitudinal and cross-sectional data offer a tantalising suggestion that the rate of loss of maximum oxygen uptake develops less rapidly in the continuing endurance athlete than in the general population'. Shephard rightly emphasises the difficulty of demonstrating conclusively that a loss of fitness can be prevented, but on the present evidence it is justifiable to encourage people to try to keep fit as they grow older as a means of preventing some of the problems that occur in old age and which were, until recently, assumed to be the result of the immutable ageing process.

The rehabilitative approach

The loss of fitness that results from the modern lifestyle can therefore be prevented, but the only effective means of prevention are sports and active leisure pursuits. The loss of fitness that is often a consequence of disabling disease is also preventable by adopting an active style of management which aims to treat not only the tissue or organ or part of the body directly affected by the pathological process but also the rest of the body which is affected by immobility. The term 'rehabilitation' is often used to mean the phase of management that follows the treatment of the causal problem, but in old age the rehabilitative approach should be used in all cases with consideration being given to the possible complications resulting from immobility as well as to the management of the disease that is causing it. One of the major contributions of geriatric medicine has been the demonstration that elderly people with disabling disease need not become heavily dependent on others provided that the disease is accurately diagnosed and effectively treated, and provided that an optimistic rehabilitative approach is adopted from the outset of treatment.

The dangers of bed rest are now appreciated (Asher, 1953; Rodahl et al, 1967; Saltin et al, 1968) but the insidious loss of fitness that results from a less specific decrease in activity is often overlooked, especially among the elderly. The importance of the rehabilitative approach is not only that it helps patients regain lost fitness but also that it prevents that loss of fitness in the first place.

CAN FITNESS BE REGAINED?

Althought this book is mainly concerned with primary and secondary prevention, it is important to review the evidence to prove that fitness can be regained in old age, in part because it has implications for the planning and management of health and social services, as will be discussed in the next section, and in part because any evidence that demonstrates older people can regain skills supports the case for prevention in old age.

The evidence that fitness can be regained in old age is not easy to assess for a number of reasons, such as the paucity of knowledge about the natural history of ageing, which makes the effectiveness of interventions difficult to asssess, and the fact that some of the important literature is written only in Russian (Gore, 1972). Nevertheless, there is now sufficient evidence to allow the conclusion to be drawn that all aspects of fitness can be regained in old age.

Regaining stamina

The results of research in the field which have been usefully summarised by Bassey (1978) are encouraging. In one study the aerobic power of 38 people age between 60 and 70 increased by 30 per cent as a result of only seven weeks' conditioning (Sidney et al, 1977) and the authors pointed out that 'maximum oxygen intake was brought quite quickly to the level anticipated in a sedentary person ten to twenty years younger than the test subject'. Another study of 112 men aged between 52 and 87 years also produced an increase in the oxygen transport capacity, due to improvements in the function of both the cardiovascular and respiratory systems and to an improvement in the efficiency of the enzymes in the muscles. (de Vries, 1970; Benestad, 1965).

Regaining strength

Recent research has confirmed that 70-year-old muscles can regain strength with training. Useful studies in Göteborg (Aniansson et al, 1980; Aniansson

& Gustafsson, 1981) have demonstrated significant increases in both static and dynamic muscular strength when a training programme was followed three times weekly for twelve weeks. Muscle biopsies were taken before and after training and microscopic examination suggested an increase in the area of Type II fibres (Figure 6.3). There is good evidence therefore that it is possible to regain strength by requiring the muscles to perform work.

Regaining suppleness

Suppleness and joint stiffness are difficult variables to measure, particularly as they change with movement. Nevertheless, in one study it was shown not only that a training programme can decrease the torque necessary to move a joint passively, but also that there may be no difference between the response of young and old subjects to the training (Chapman et al, 1972) (Table 6.5). In another study, a thrice-weekly exercise and dance programme, continued for twelve weeks, produced a significant increase in movement at six sites — neck, wrist, shoulder, hip and back, knee and ankle (Munns, 1981).

Regaining skill

Even a developing brain can lose skills, as anyone who has observed the effect

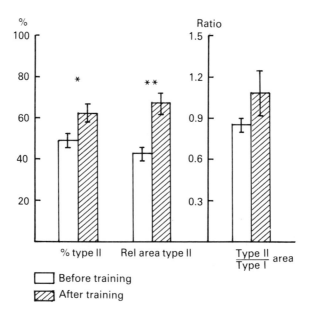

Fig. 6.3 Relative number and relative area of type II fibres and ratio between the mean fibre area of Type II and Type I fibres in the right vastus lateralis before and after training in 69-74-year-old men ($n = 9$). Mean and SE are given, * and ** denote $P<0.05$ and $P<0.01$ respectively (Aniansson & Gustafsson, 1981)

Table 6.5 Effect of training on torque necessary to move index finger passively about metacarpophalangeal joint (Chapman et al, 1972)

	Pre-training		Post-training	
	Mean	SE	Mean	SE
Young				
Experimental	1.458	0.104	1.148	0.097*
Control	1.291	0.087	1.183	0.076
Old				
Experimental	2.166	0.235	1.709	0.123*
Control	2.144	0.168	1.931	0.145

*Significance of pre-post difference, $p<0.05$ Torque is measured in Kg-Cm

that lack of practice can have on the piano-playing skills of a ten-year-old will attest. The ageing brain loses the ability to perform complicated actions if those skills are not practised, and in old age this can have very serious repercussions because the skills that are lost may be those that are essential for daily living, for example the skill of putting an arm in a sleeve, or the skill of pulling one's pants up.

There is also evidence that those who remain active do not experience so great an increase in their reaction times as those who become inactive as they grow older (Sherwood & Selder, 1979) (Fig. 6.4). The authors are cautious in their interpretation of their results but the difference between the two groups is striking and obviously requires more research. An even more interesting study, conducted in the Soviet Union, cited in Gore's review of the Russian literature (Gore, 1972), was one in which a small number of people were followed for ten years during which time they performed daily exercise, and participated in two ninety-minute group exercise sessions. There was improvement, most marked after three years, in many aspects of fitness including their coordination and balance, and the majority of the subjects were able to stand for a longer period of time with their eyes shut after the period of training (Gore, 1972). There is thus evidence that the control and coordination of movements which develops during childhood and adolescence but declines in old age can be improved by training in old age.

The general conclusion that may be drawn from research is, therefore, encouraging (Shephard, 1978; Smith & Serfass, 1981). There is obviously a need for more research, notably for intervention studies in which elderly people, both fit elderly people and those suffering from chronic disease, are randomly allocated either to fitness programmes or to control situations, but the need for more research should not delay the implementation of the research findings that are already available.

PSYCHOLOGICAL BENEFITS OF EXERCISE

To the physical benefits of exercise can be added psychological benefits. The

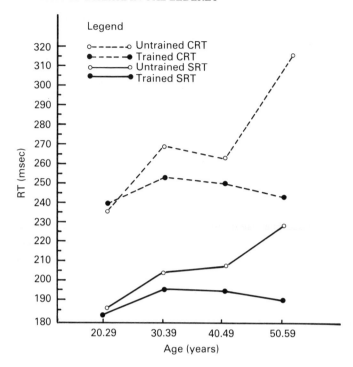

Fig. 6.4 The relationship of reaction time, age and fitness level. (SRT = simple reaction time; CRT = choice reaction time) (Sherwood & Selder, 1979)

benefit most commonly enjoyed by old people who take exercise is an enhanced feeling of wellbeing. More specifically, studies have shown that elderly people who enter a ten-week exercise programme feel less anxious (Fig. 6.5) (Blumenthal & Williams, 1982).

The mechanisms by which exercise reduces anxiety and increases wellbeing have not yet been precisely identified but the effects are consistently demonstrated.

RISKS OF EXERCISE IN OLD AGE

There is no evidence that the encouragement of older people to take more exercise will result in a significant mortality. Isometric exercise is dangerous, but the most hazardous forms of isometric exercise in middle and old age are not encountered in active leisure activities. They are more likely to occur in daily life, for example when pushing a car on a cold morning or hurrying across the airport terminal carrying a heavy suitcase. Isotonic exercise may be hazardous, because it has been suggested that an increasingly active lifestyle in old age is, in part, responsible for the increasing incidence of fractured

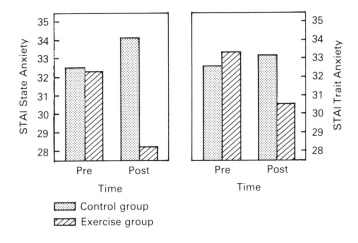

Fig. 6.5 Comparison of exercise and control group scores on state (left) and trait (right) anxiety before and after the ten-week exercise programme (Blumenthal & Williams, 1982)

neck of femur that has been observed in the United Kingdom, but this is, at present, only a hypothesis.

It is possible that older people are at an increased risk of soft tissue injuries, but many such injuries can be prevented if the old person is not simply exhorted to take more exercise but is given instruction on the types of exercise that are most suitable for older people, the need to warm up when taking exercise, and the importance of changing from an inactive to a more active lifestyle gradually rather than abruptly.

IMPLICATIONS FOR SERVICE PLANNING

Implications for health educators

Inactivity is a major risk factor in old age, and the promotion of enjoyable activity should therefore form a central theme in any health education programme. However, elderly people need to be listened to before they are talked at, for it is essential to hear their beliefs about, and attitudes towards, exercise in old age before offering advice or prescribing exercise (McHeath, 1984).

The type of advice that people need is not vague exhortations to take more exercise but specific information about the intensity, frequency and duration of exercise which is necessary to improve their level of fitness. This should be combined with suggestions as to the type of exercise they might find enjoyable, together with information on the availability of leisure facilities and the offer of assistance for those who are unable to reach their local facilities because they have limited mobility. In addition, many older people welcome information about the safety of exercise and the steps that can be taken to reduce any risk.

The needs of active elderly people, housebound elderly people and the institutionalised elderly vary, and a different approach is required for each group. The more active elderly people take enough exercise to maintain strength and stamina, but few take specific action to prevent loss of suppleness, and the recommendation that they try swimming or yoga or music and movement is often relevant. Housebound elderly people may also be working so hard that they are maintaining their strength and stamina simply by looking after themselves, as J. B. Priestley eloquently describes:

> Why not a piece, as honest as I can make it on Old Age? A lot of people have told us how they are enjoying — or have enjoyed — their old age. I am not one of these complacent ancients. I detest being old. I can't settle down to make the most of it — whatever that may be — but resent almost every aspect of it...Because I am old, almost everything demands both effort and patience. Nothing runs itself. What — even getting dressed or going to bed? Certainly. They are both workouts. I do not say tremendous efforts are involved, but there are no easy routines here, nothing accomplished while thinking about something else. I can have a little wrestling match just getting into a pair of trousers. Just coping with the mere arrangements of ordinary living, there must continually be an exercise of will. To get by from nine in the morning until midnight I use enough will power to command an army corps.

Some disabled elderly people, however, work so slowly, stopping to rest frequently, that they continue to lose fitness even though they remain active, albeit at a slower rate than would be the case if they were to stop caring for themselves and rely on others to do so. The reason that some disabled elderly people stop as soon as they feel distressed obviously varies from one individual to another. Some believe that their bodies will be harmed if they become breathless, while others simply find the effort so daunting that they prefer to divide it into a series of small steps. It is worthwhile telling disabled people that they will benefit if they do housework with sufficient vigour to increase their pulse and respiratory rates, but the appeal of such an argument is limited. Housework is of limited appeal at the best of times, to the newly-wed bride for example, and to people who have been doing housework and looking after themselves for decades the exhortation to perform household tasks with more vigour will, understandably, be received with little enthusiasm.

Housebound people are in even greater need of the stimulation that new forms of exercise and company offer than those elders who are active, mobile elderly people. It is often difficult to arrange for housebound old people to participate in enjoyable activities sufficiently, often because of the shortage of transport to day or leisure centres, and for this reason attempts should be made to encourage activity in the home, and because housework and self-care do not provide sufficient stimulus to maintain suppleness, even if done with sufficient vigour to maintain strength and stamina, it is appropriate to teach elderly people simple exercises to maintain and improve suppleness. Shoulder stiffness is a common and disabling problem in old age because housework and self-care make relatively few demands on the rotator cuff muscles. Simple rotatory movements can therefore be helpful, provided that they are performed daily.

Institutionalised old people are in some ways more fortunate than disabled people in their own homes, for example because they may have organised physical activity classes in the home, but in other ways they may be relatively disadvantaged, notably because the old person in her own home usually has to struggle more than the old person in residential care for whom the style of care that is provided all too often results in a loss of many of the activities and decisions that formerly kept the individual fit and active. The provision of physiotherapy or physical activity several times weekly cannot compensate for the loss of the physiotherapy and occupational therapy of daily life, and if disabled elderly people are to be helped to maintain and improve their fitness, it is essential that they be offered not only health education but also a style of service that will not increase their disability and unfitness.

Implications for the caring services

Rehabilitation is too often considered to be a distinct type of management provided by specialists such as occupational and physiotherapists. This is, however, an inappropriate concept because only a proportion of disabled people are ever treated by specialist rehabilitation services. The majority are managed by general practitioners and community nurses, and it is essential that the rehabilitative approach should be more frequently used by the those professionals than is the case at present. Too often the elderly person who has developed a problem with self-care, difficulty with cooking or housework for example, is simply prescribed a prosthesis such as meals on wheels or a home help instead of being given a comprehensive assessment and the appropriate form of treatment to help her regain the skill. In part this occurs because there are insufficient physiotherapists and occupational therapists working outside hospital, but it is not simply due to shortage of resources. General practitioners and community nurses need to take a more rehabilitative approach to the problems of elderly people, based on a functional assessment with practical advice on the problems of daily living and with clear and specific prescriptions for exercise as a complement to and, in some cases, a substitute for a prescription of medication.

An even greater problem exists in the personal social services which are considered to be providers of 'care' rather than 'treatment', because 'care' is too often interpreted as meaning that everything possible should be done for an old person who is having difficulty. Consider, for example, an old lady who is having increasing difficulty in preparing food because of her arthritis. She is visited by her niece who lives far away and who sees her infrequently.

The niece is concerned to see her aunt struggling to peel potatoes and prepare lunch. She tells her aunt to sit and rest while she prepares lunch, and then refers her aunt for meals on wheels which will be provided if there is spare capacity in the meals on wheels service.

Such a sequence of event happens frequently, not only because of the shortage of occupational therapists in social services departments but also because the expectations of both the applicants and the providers of social services are that need will be met with care, and by 'care' is meant the provision of services that perform the skill that is lost. Those services may be considered to be prostheses for the replacement of a loss of function as a wheelchair replaces the loss of the ability to walk. Prostheses which are prescribed without appropriate assessment accelerate the rate at which fitness is lost.

The design of the physical environment can also accelerate the rate of loss of fitness. For example, the provision of lifts in a two-storey block of flats obviously helps those tenants who find it impossible to climb stairs to a first floor, but the availability of the lift has adverse effects on those first-floor tenants who can climb stairs but who use a lift if one is available. It would be better not to provide lifts but to design the stairs so that an elderly person could sit and rest halfway, housing in a ground-floor flat those who found the ascent very difficult or impossible. In this way the majority would be encouraged to remain active and preserve their fitness. Similarly, the control of heating in old people's flats at a central point and the inclusion of a standard heating charge in the rent, as opposed to individual control by each tenant, certainly reduces the risks of hypothermia, but it also reduces the number of decisions and calculations that the elderly tenants are required to make and this also reduces their fitness.

Attitudes to care

The attitudes that prevail in most societies are responsible for this type of care, a type of care which overprotects and underestimates elderly people. The attitudes symbolised by, and expressed through, this type of care derive in part from the belief that all the problems of old people result from the immutable ageing process, but they are also a consequence of guilt. Many younger people are concerned about the position of elderly people in society but prefer to make token gestures, for example by doing simple jobs for elderly people, by paying others to do such tasks, rather than providing elderly people with the resources to do things for themselves. They do this to relieve their own guilt as well as to help the old person.

The attitudes and beliefs of old people are also important. Some old people believe that rest is therapeutic, others that it is pointless trying to prevent the disabilities that they believe are all caused by 'old age', namely the ageing process. Some old people have the understandable attitude that it is their right to have things done for them after decades of toil. This attitude is particularly strong among those elderly people who are paying for the care they receive, for most pay more for residential care than they ever paid for their most luxurious holiday and such an attitude is, in many people, further reinforced if they see other old people receiving the same type of care even though they are not paying for it. In a local authority home for old people in the United Kingdom, residents who have saved and who thus have capital pay £100 per week, whereas residents who have no savings are supported by the State, yet each sees the other receive exactly the same services. The tension is further increased if the old person who pays knows the biography of the person who does not have to pay, as often happens in homes which serve discrete communities; it is all too easy for the old person who is paying to classify the old person who is not as being less deserving, for example because he drank or was often unemployed or never saved enough to buy a house. In such circumstances the suggestion that the old person should do more for herself is unlikely to be met with enthusiasm and may be received with frank hostility

Inactivity may be encouraged by staff, either because the staff member likes the gratitude that results from the performance of a task for an old person or, more commonly, because staffing levels are too low to allow the staff to foster independence, for it is often faster to perform tasks for disabled old person than it is to allow them a perform them for themselves. Low staffing levels can also create dependence, because the old person who is being cared for soon learns that an improvement in her functional ability will lead to a reduction in the number of contacts with staff, if she is in a home, or in the number of visits from her home help or district nurse if she is in her own home.

FUTURE PATTERNS

The growth in the amount of evidence demonstrating the beneficial effects of exercise in old age has coincided with the growth of public interest, and participation, in active leisure pursuits. The cohorts who will reach old age in the future will have more positive beliefs about, and attitudes towards, exercise than the cohorts who are old today. They will, hopefully, also be advised by professionals who are more aware of the benefits of exercise than today's professionals (see page 89). It is probable therefore that exercise promotion will play a much more prominent part in the delivery of health and social services in future than it does today.

REFERENCES

Aniansson A, Grimby G, Rundgren A, Svanborg A, Orlander J 1980 Physical training in old men. Age and Ageing 9: 186–187

Aniansson A, Grimby G, Hedberg M, Krotkiewki M 1981 Muscle morphology, enzyme activity and muscle strength in elderly men and women. Clinical Physiology, 1: 73–86

Aniansson A, Gustafsson E 1981 Physical training in elderly men with special reference to quadriceps muscle strength and morphology. Clinical Physiology 1:87-98

Asher R 1947 The dangers of going to bed. British Medical Journal 2: 967–968

Astrand P, Rodahl K 1971 Textbook of work physiology: physiological bases of exercise, 2nd edn. McGraw Hill, New York

Bassey E J 1978 Age, inactivity and some physiological responses to exercise. Gerontology 24: 66–77

Benestad A M 1965 Trainability of older men. Acta Medica Scandinavica 178: 321–327

Blumenthal J A, Williams, R S 1982 Advances in Research, 6:3. Duke University Centre for the Study of Aging and Human Development

Chapman E A, de Vries H A, Swezcy R 1972 Joint stiffness: effects of exercise on young and old men. Journal of Gerontology 27: 218–221

de Vries H A 1970 Physiological effects of an exercise training regime upon men aged 52 to 88. Journal of Gerontology 25: 325–336

Gore I Y 1972 Physical activity and ageing — a survey of the Russian literature. Gerontologia Clinica 14: 65–85

Gray J A M 1982 Practising prevention in old age. British Medical Journal 285: 545–7

Lewis A F 1981 Fracture of neck of the femur: changing incidence. British Medical Journal 2: 1217–1219

MacHealth J A 1984 Activity, health and fitness in old age. Croom Helm, London

Munns K 1981 Effects of exercise on the range of joint motion in elderly patients. In: Smith B L, Serfass R C (eds). Exercise and Aging. (Enslow, p 167–178

Rodahl K, Birkhead N C, Blizzard J J Issekutz B, Pruett E D R 1967 Nutrition and physical activity. Symposium of the Swedish Nutrition Foundation

Saltin B, Bloaquist G, Mitchell J H, Johnson R L, Wildenthal K, Chapman C B 1968 Response to exercise after bedrest and after training. Circulation 38 (Suppl 7): 1–51

Shephard R J 1978 Physical activity and aging. Croom Helm, New York

Sherwood, D E and Selder, D S 1979 Cardiorespiratory health, reaction time and aging. Medicine and Science in Sports 11: 168–169

Sidney K H, Shephard R J, Harrison J E 1977 Endurance training and body composition of the elderly. American Journal of Nutrition 30: 326–333

Smith E L, and Serfass R C (eds) 1981 Exercise and ageing: the scientific basis. Enslow

7

Robert Lindsay

Prevention of osteoporosis

INTRODUCTION

Osteoporosis is a disorder of ageing which is rapidly becoming a major public health problem in many countries. Treatment, once the disorder is clinically manifest, is difficult, and prevention may offer the best solution to this major clinical problem for the elderly. However, when considering the approaches to prevention of osteoporosis, it is important to understand clearly the aims for such a program. Ultimately, the goal must be reduction in the incidence of those fractures which are the clinical expression of the disorder. It is generally held that fractures in osteoporosis result, at least partially, because the skeleton has attained a sufficiently weakened status such that even a trivial injury will cause the bone to break. It is clearly obvious that if prevention is to be effective, it must not only prevent the skeletal deterioration which precedes fracture occurrence, but must also take cognizance of those factors which will precipitate the traumatic incident and attempt to eliminate, or at least reduce, their incidence. Thus, predisposing factors which lead to falls and other causes of trivial trauma among the elderly are an important issue in preventive aspects of fracture among the elderly (see Ch. 9).

This chapter is concerned only with the phenomenon of bone loss with ageing in the adult human, and the role of the reduced bone mass in the pathophysiology of fractures among the elderly. It will explore our capability to identify those individuals who may be at risk from the disease, at an age when preventive therapy might be successfully instituted. It will also examine the evidence that prevention of bone loss can be successfully undertaken, with some attention to the costs and benefits to be obtained from such an approach.

Definition

Osteoporosis is a disorder in which reduction of bone tissue per unit volume of anatomical bone sufficiently compromises the skeleton such that fractures may occur on minimal or trivial trauma.

THE DISEASE

While some authorities would not accept the presence of the disorder osteoporosis until fracture has occurred, and prefer to use the word osteopenia for the reduction in bone mass, this is an exercise in semantics. After the skeleton has become compromised by sufficient loss of bone, fracture occurrence is only a matter of time and circumstance. The basic pathophysiology does not change following the fracture incident.

Histologically, the bone exhibits both osteoporosity and osteopenia. The introduction of techniques allowing accurate estimation of bone mass permits the diagnosis of reduced skeletal mass, even in the absence of fracture. Such a situation might be called, more correctly, asymptomatic or subclinical osteoporosis. These non-invasive techniques for bone mass measurement also allow identification of individuals who are losing bone at a comparatively rapid rate, within a reasonable time frame (three months to a year). In this fashion, for younger asymptomatic patients, measurement of both bone mineral mass and rate of loss will allow some determination of risk. Such techniques do not identify the mechanisms involved in bone loss but merely its presence. They do, however, allow intervention and the institution of preventive measures at a significantly earlier stage than has previously been the case. In addition, there is an accompanying increased potential for success, since the skeletal changes following therapy can be monitored in a relatively accurate fasion.

In addition, it has been evident for some time that no techniques exist which will allow us, using bone mass measurements alone, to separate patients with osteoporotic fractures from so-called 'normal' individuals (Fig. 7.1). Even the most sophisticated techniques show at least a 40 per cent

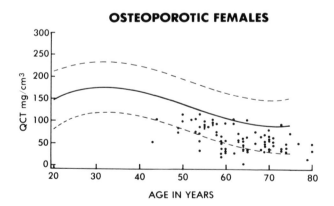

Fig. 7.1 Bone mass as a function of age in a normal population. Solid line indicates the mean; and dotted lines, 95% confidence limits. Measurements are made by quantitative computerised axial tomography of trabecular bone in the lumbar vertebral body. The patients with osteoporosis (●) almost all lie within normal volumes for age, but are generally below the norm value (From Genant et al, 1983, with permission).

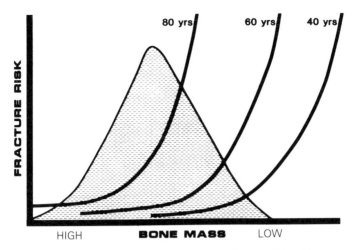

Fig. 7.2 A graphic description of the relationship between fracture risk and bone mass, both of which change as a function of age. As the normal distribution of bone mass falls with age and fracture risk increases, there is an increasing overlap of the two phenomena with increasing age.

overlap with the normal population, although most of the patient group fall below the 50th percentile for the population; that is to say that 40 per cent of 'osteoporotic' fractures occur in individuals who by bone mass estimation are normal; or, alternatively, normal individuals over 60 years whose bone mass is below average for their age and sex must be considered to be at risk from fracture.

This relationship between fracture risk and bone mass at any age can be demonstrated graphically (Fig. 7.2), showing the continuum of fracture risk which overlaps normal bone range, and increasingly so with age as bone mass falls. High risk of fracture is therefore a 'normal' expectation for many older individuals and results from the bone loss which inevitably accompanies ageing. Prevention of bone loss should result in only a significant reduction of the expected shift to the left of the fracture risk line as age progresses. If bone loss were to be completely inhibited, then any shift in the line would result from the increased tendency of the elderly to fall.

The relative importance of these two influences on fracture risk (bone mass and frequency of falls) cannot be determined at present. What is clear is that those fractures which are considered to result from the disease osteoporosis are rapidly becoming a major public health problem, which must be tackled by preventive methods.

The scope of the problem

It has been realised for many years that overall fracture incidence increases with age and that the rise in fracture incidence occurs earlier and is greater among women than men (Gallagher et al, 1980). More recently it has become generally accepted that loss of bone with age is a universal phenomenon which can be observed from the third or fourth decade in both men and women (Cann, 1980). Some studies have suggested a linear reduction in bone mineral greater in women than in men (Riggs et al, 1982). Others have suggested an acceleration of bone loss around or after the time of the menopause in women with a subsequent, somewhat exponential decline in bone loss thereafter (Hui et al, 1982).

Fractures resulting from osteoporosis are significantly more common in women than in men (approximately eight fractures in women for every fracture among males). Maximum bone mass in women is somewhat less at maturity and subsequent bone loss greater. It is likely, therefore, that by age 60 years bone mass has been reduced through some theoretical fracture threshold in at least 25 per cent of all women.

Epidemiological data are difficult to obtain for osteoporosis, but it has been suggested that these 25 per cent of women who have developed a compromised skeleton by the age of 60 years will, in fact, have radiological evidence of osteoporosis. In the United States, by the end of the next decade, more than five million women of the twenty million over the age of 65 years would, therefore, have radiological evidence of the disorder. The number of such women who will develop fractures of clinical significance is difficult to predict. However, some studies suggest that, of all women who reach the age of 80 years, one in four will have had a hip fracture, and indeed the incidence of hip fracture in the population doubles by each decade after 50 years (Gordan & Vaughn, 1976). The overall incidence of fractures of the proximal femur are approximately 1.3 per cent per annum for the female population over the age of 65 and about 0.3 per cent per annum for males over the age of 65 (Lindsay, unpublished observation). The real incidence of vertebral crush fractures, the most common osteoporotic fracture, is unknown, since this fracture by itself does not usually result in hospital admission.

Using fractures of the proximal femur as the benchmark, recent evidence indicates that the overall incidence of the disorder is increasing. Data from centres in the United Kingdom and the USA have suggested that hospital admissions and discharges as a result of fractures of the femoral neck are increasing every decade at a rate greater than would be expected from the rise in the medium age of the population (Fenton-Lewis, 1982; Lindsay & Herrington, 1983; Wallace, 1983.) Our own data generated from discharge data obtained from a cross-sectional survey of the United States indicates a rise in incidence of both vertebral fracture and hip fracture. About 60 per cent of the increment can be accounted for by the increasing median age of the population and, therefore, the increased absolute numbers of individuals at risk.

Presently, in 1984 we expect in excess of three hundred thousand hip fractures in the United States (both intertrochanteric and sub-capital fractures), and by the end of the century, if the current increase continues, there will be approximately 0.5 million fractures per year in the USA.

Not only hip fractures result in a considerable fiscal drain in terms of health care costs (Fig. 7.3.) but also a significant morbidity and mortality. The total cost of health care for fractures of the hip in the United States is somewhere in excess of $4 million currently and may quadruple by the end of the century. In most studies, in which hip fracture patients have been observed, there is an associated mortality of approximately 10 per cent (Jensen & Tondevold, 1979). Such mortality figures would bring hip fracture into the top twelve or so most common causes of death in the United States. In addition, about 30 per cent of the patients admitted to acute hospitals as a result of hip fracture are subsequently discharged to long-term care institutions, placing a further burden on the health care delivery systems.

PREVENTIVE THERAPY

It has proved difficult to provide therapy for patients with clinically overt osteoporosis which would raise bone mass sufficiently for the risk of recurring fracture to be significantly reduced. Many techniques have been invoked by physicians in an attempt to do this; most have failed. Early prevention of bone loss seems the most rational approach that might result in significant fracture prevention among the older population. Indeed, one may expect that if *successful* regimes of preventive therapy can be instituted over a sufficiently long period of time, then there must be a dramatic reduction in fracture incidence. How great this reduction could or would be, particularly when one considers fractures of the hip, is unknown. The tendency to fall, which increases with age, will ensure that fractures will continue to occur among the elderly despite increased bone strength.

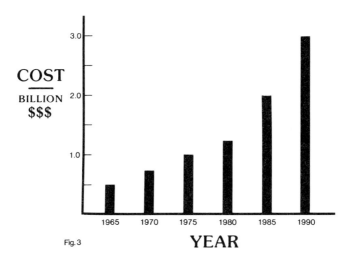

Fig. 7.3 The cost of acute-health care for fracture of the neck of the femur in the USA for 1965 through 1990.

The issues that confront professionals concerned about prevention are as follows:
1. To whom preventive therapy should be provided — the 'at-risk' population
2. Which forms of preventive therapy are most effective in retarding bone loss
3. When intervention should begin
4. How long therapy should continue to afford effective prevention.

Identification of individuals at risk

For prevention to be successful, it is clear that we must develop a method for identification of individuals at risk at a point when intervention is possible. The sexual dimorphism in *skeletal mass* appears at adolescence, with the greater growth spurt and the development of significantly larger muscle mass in males (Garn, 1970). In addition, at least in prior years, the participation of males in more vigorous exercise pursuits may have played a role in establishing greater skeletal mass, a factor which may be of lesser importance among young people of today. However, by early adulthood it is already clear that women are already liable to be more at risk of osteoporosis than men.

Bone loss after maturity in the third decade in life is a universal phenomenon analogous to the loss of lean body mass with age (Garn, 1970; Riggs et al, 1981). This relationship between muscle mass and skeletal mass may account, at least in part, for the racial differences in skeletal mass, as well as the differences between the sexes. It is, however, mostly after the menopause in the female that the sexual dichotomy in *bone loss* becomes most obvious. Oestrogen deficiency is followed by a twofold increment in bone turnover (Heaney, Recker & Saville, 1978a) and a period of loss of trabecular bone, which may reach 5–10 per cent per annum in trabecular bone (Cann et al, 1980). For this reason, among others, the time of menopause is a useful marker to attempt to identify women at risk, although *some* preventive advice can and should be offered to the younger population.

Since we cannot, nor should we attempt to, offer 'blanket' therapy for the entire female population, it is important to categorise those individuals particularly at risk, at the time of menopause at the latest. Certain clinical associations have been described for those patients who present with clinical disease, and currently the physician can use these to attempt to identify high-risk individuals at an early age (Table 7.1).

Clinical osteoporosis is clearly a disorder which occurs predominantly in women. It is common among those of Caucasian and Asiatic ethnic derivation, but is of much lower incidence among blacks. When a family history can be obtained from patients with established disease, then almost 90 per cent will be positive for this disorder among mother, grandmother, or aunts. Osteoporosis classically occurs among slim women (Saville, 1970). In his original description of the disease, Albright (1940) delineated the importance

Table 7.1 Risk factors for osteoporosis

1. Females of white or oriental origin
2. Positive family history for osteoporosis
3. Poor diet, including: – low calcium intake
   – high caffeine intake
   – high protein intake
   – high phosphate intake
4. Early menopause or oophorectomy
5. Sedentary lifestyle
6. Reduced weight for height
7. Alcohol abuse
8. Cigarette smoking
9. Nulliparity

of an early menopause or oophorectomy, facts which are still regarded as probably among the most important. Indeed, as we have said, the very presence of a menopause among the female of the species may be the crucial factor in the sexual dichotomy exhibited by the incidence of osteoporotic fractures.

The major remaining risk factors can be divided into dietary and lifestyle factors, and therefore are potentially correctable. Of the dietary factors, insufficient intake of calcium is probably the most important, but association between high caffeine, protein and phosphate intakes and disease incidence have been suggested. A high alcohol intake neatly links dietary and lifestyle factors. Although osteoporosis is clearly associated with alcoholic liver disease (Saville, 1965), it is also evidence that a high alcohol intake without overt hepatic dysfunction is clinically commonly associated with osteoporosis occurring at a young age, or osteoporosis among males (Seeman et al, 1983). A sedentary lifestyle also appears to be of great importance, and associations between osteoporosis and cigarette smoking have been reported (Daniell, 1976; Lindsay, 1981). The role of nulliparity is not clear, although a theoretical argument for this being a risk factor can be made. However, nulliparity is not nearly as evident when one examines these risk factors in a clinical setting. Finally, the existence of intercurrent disease processes affecting mineral metabolism, such as thyrotoxicosis, hyperparathyroidism, Cushing's disease, and diabetes mellitus, will clearly exacerbate the problem.

Despite the ready description of such associations, it is difficult for the clinician to know the weight which should be given to each of these 'risk' factors when he/she is faced with a young patient wishing advice about prevention. In addition, the possible additive or even synergistic effect of these factors when several are present in one individual is not understood.

The use of bone mass measurement

Now that non-invasive techniques for estimating bone mineral mass are becoming increasingly available, it may be that screening techniques in the future should involve both these clinical risk factors already enumerated and bone mass measurements. The techniques (Table 7.2) which are available vary enormously in capital expense and cost to the patient, as well as accuracy and reproducibility, and they have been described in detail in the recent literature (Mazess, 1979; Dequeker & Johnson, 1981).

Currently, our laboratory utilises both dual-and single-beam photon absorptiometry. The combination of these techniques allows us estimates of both peripheral (mid or distal radius) and central (lumbar vertebrae, or neck of femur) sites. The bone measured is primarily cortical at the peripheral sites and is a combination of both trabecular and cortical bone at the central sites. Whichever techniques are adopted, it is critical to obtain not only normative data but also good estimates of the accuracy and precision of the technique, appropriate to the particular clinic setting, since estimates, particularly of precision, may vary significantly for each technique and are often operator-dependent.

The most common technique available at present is single-photon absorptiometry. However, recent evidence suggesting that changes occurring centrally may differ from those occurring at the periphery (Riggs et al, 1981) makes it imperative for those who wish to use such techniques to have available both a central and a peripheral estimate. A combination of techniques involving measurements of radial and lumbar vertebral mineral using single-and dual-photon techniques produces a radiation exposure equal to that obtained from a single chest X-ray and may be, under well-controlled circumstances, both accurate and sufficiently reproducible to allow follow-up of individual patients. Relatively modest capital investment and running costs also make this combination of techniques attractive. For those who have access to computerised axial tomography (CAT scan), this technique pro-

Table 7.2 Non-invasive techniques for measurement of bone mass

Technique	Site	Cortical/trabecular ratio	Accuracy (%)	Precision (%)	Radiation
Radiogrammetry	Metacarpal	99:1	?	±2	5–8 mrem
Radiodensitometry	Metacarpal	99:1	?	2–15	5–8 mrem
Single-photon absorptiometry	Mid-radius	95:5	4	2–4	5 mrem
	Distal radius	75:25	5	2–4	5 mrem
Dual-photon absorptiometry	LV 2–4	40:60	5–7	2–5	5–15 mrem
	Femur neck	75:25	?	?	5–15 mrem
	Total skeleton	80:20	2–4	2–4	10–40 mrem
Computerised tomography	Vertebral body	5:95	?*	?*	>200 mrem
Neutron activation analysis	Total body	80:20	3–5	2–3	>1 rem
	Trunk	30:70	±10	5	400 mrem

*Precision and accuracy of CT vary depending on methodology — dual energy scanning improves accuracy (by some correction for marrow fat), but precision does not appear to change. Radiation dosage doubles, however.

PREVENTION OF OSTEOPOROSIS 103

vides, with appropriate software, accurate estimates of trabecular bone, unobtainable by other techniques (Genant et al, 1983).

The CAT scan technique allows sampling of pure trabecular bone within the vertebral body (Fig. 7.4) and, using an appropriate dual energy technique, will allow at least some correction for fat which replaces resorbed bone.

Practically, it would be useful to have some estimate of bone turnover which could be easily performed within the clinic setting, since turnover is likely to be related to the rate of bone loss. Using such a technique in combination with a mass estimate might give a more reliable 'risk estimate'. Additionally, all investigations could be performed at one clinic visit, obviating the need for repeated estimates of bone mass over a period of time before bone loss is documented for each individual. We have developed a quantitative technique for the standard bone scan which gives a reasonable estimate of bone turnover and may be useful in the clinical setting (Fogelman et al, 1980).

For patients worried about bone loss and its prevention, the capability to achieve a quick answer is clearly advantageous. However, currently bone mass measurements are available only in specialised centres, and estimates of bone turnover are virtually unavailable. Therefore, the clinician often has to rely on the presence or absence of the so-called 'risk factors' to make a judgement about prevention.

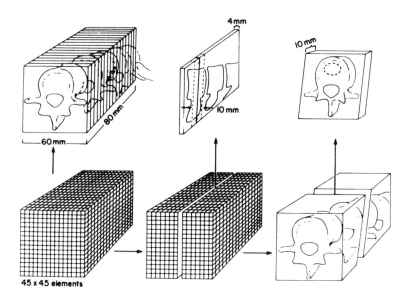

Fig. 7.4 Diagrammatic representation of image reconstruction techniques used to obtain a 'pure' sample of trabecular bone from the vertebral body (From Genant et al, 1983, with permission).

Provision of preventive therapy

Having arrived at some conclusion for each individual patient, based on the data obtained using the related clinical phenomena, plus perhaps bone mass estimations, the clinician is faced with a decision about intervention with preventive therapy. There are currently no hard-and-fast rules which can be followed, and we must consider the following questions: For which of the at-risk groups of patients should physicians provide intervention therapy? Which forms of preventive therapy are effective, and for how long should they be provided?

To resolve these problems in a preliminary fashion, until more scientific data are available, we have established the following criteria for the use of preventive measures. If available, we use bone mass estimations to determine necessity for prevention. If bone mass is low (<33 percentile of our normal population), preventive measures are instituted. If bone mass is normal, but repeat estimates confirm a significant downward trend (i.e., greater than or equal to the 'normal' downward trend), preventive steps are begun at that point. The presence of 'clinical osteoporosis' requires treatment, not prevention. Where such techniques are not available, the presence of *one* of *three* major clinical associations is sufficient to consider preventive efforts.

1. Poor diet — calcium intake normally < 500 g
   — high alcohol intake
2. Poor lifestyle — cigarette smoker
   — sedentary lifestyle
   (expenditure < 500 kcal/day)
3. Early menopause or oophorectomy

Clearly, the first two are items that are correctable by the patients themselves; remediation for the third requires physician intervention.

Calcium

For many years, a poor calcium diet has been considered to be an important factor in the pathogenesis of osteoporosis. Several observations suggest that the human species consumes a diet generally calcium-deficient. Support comes from teleological studies which show that the human species consumes a diet significantly lower in calcium (per unit body weight) than that of most other mammals (Heaney, Recker & Saville, 1977). The Hanes studies in the USA confirmed the low calcium intake (for an adult, approximately 10 mg/kg/day while the recommended daily intake is 800 mg/day (or 16 mg/kg/day for the average woman). Heaney (1965), in attempting a unifying hypothesis for the pathogenesis of osteoporosis, proposed that the central problem was this low calcium intake throughout adult life, which by itself could explain the role of other 'pathogenetic' influences.

More recent elegant studies from the same laboratory (Heaney, Recker & Saville, 1978b) showed a deficit of 20 mg/calcium/day in premenopausal women, rising to 40 mg/day in postmenopausal women. These values equate to total mineral losses of 1/2 per cent per annum in premenopausal women and one per cent per annum among postmenopausal women, figures somewhat similar to those obtained from cross-sectional data of bone mineral measurements performed on cortical bone, and from our own longitudinal data (Lindsay et al, 1980). It has been suggested, therefore, that premenopausal women would *on average* be in calcium balance if obtaining the recommended daily intake of 800 mg/day. The changes which occur in postmenopausal women have been interpreted as indicative of decreased efficiency in calcium utilisation such that, to obtain calcium balance, an average intake of about 1.5 g/day would be required.

However, the most convincing evidence of the importance of calcium comes from the data of Matkovic et al (1979). In this study, fracture incidence was compared in two villages in Yugoslavia, one of which had a relatively high endogenous calcium intake (about 940/day) and the other a calcium intake closer to American standards (441 mg/day). A dramatic reduction in fracture incidence was observed in the high-calcium district, suggesting that lifelong high calcium intake would prevent the fracture increase with age. Determinations of bone mineral content by radiogrammetry indicated that, in the high-calcium district, the bone mass at maturity was greater than in the low-calcium district. Curiously, subsequent rates of bone loss appeared to be slightly *greater* in the high-calcium district, and the average bone mass measurements were almost equal by the age of 70 years. Thus, those results might suggest that calcium could not be used as an intervention therapy in mid-life.

Three studies have directly examined prevention with calcium supplementation in a prospective fashion. Two of those studies (Recker, Saville & Heaney, 1977; Horsman et al, 1977) showed reduction in bone loss when calcium intake was increased to about 1–1/2 g/day. However, recent data from Christiansen et al (1980) failed to find any effect on bone loss utilising supplemental calcium, although it must be pointed out that their patient population come from an area with a high endogenous calcium intake. Therefore, while there is no doubt that calcium deficiency is an important pathogenetic factor, it is still unclear whether or not calcium supplementation by itself will prevent the disease if given in sufficient quantities for a long period. In addition, the long-term risks or other potential benefits of a high calcium intake have yet to be evaluated.

Exercise

Recent studies have indicated that abnormal situations of inactivity, such as prolonged bed rest and exposure to zero gravity, will result in excessive loss of bone mass. However, it does not follow from the observations that large or small increases in exercise for the 'normally active' population will be necessarily beneficial. In examples of high activity, marathon runners have been shown to have higher skeletal mass (Aloia et al, 1978), and among other athletes, local skeletal mass is greater in the most frequently used limb (Montoye et al, 1980).

Additionally, several studies have now suggested that exercise programmes of comparatively short duration may influence bone mineral mass. Walking and running exercises (one hour, twice weekly) significantly increased bone mass of the lumbar spine (Krolner et al, 1983), and somewhat similar programmes have also been shown to be effective (Aloia, Cohn & Ostuni, 1978; Smith, Reddan & Smith, 1981). However, in our own preliminary observations, physical activity appears important as a determinant of bone mass only when there is a sufficiently high calcium intake to produce a positive calcium balance. Also, exercise programmes of sufficient severity to result in amenorrhoea in women may be detrimental to skeletal health.

Thus, we feel that there is still some doubt about the usefulness of physical activity by itself for prevention of bone loss. However, we recommend moderate physical activity to everyone who has no medical contra-indication, on basic good health principles. In general, for our younger patients, we follow the guidelines for exercise for good cardiovascular health, usually a minimum of 20–30 minutes of vigorous aerobic exercise on alternative days. If time permits, this can easily be supplemented by increased walking, climbing stairs, etc. Walking may be the only exercise suitable for more elderly patients, except perhaps swimming. Since it appears that rate of change of force may be more important than the absolute size of the force used, competitive racquet sports may be beneficial if played vigorously. However, individuals over 35 years who are beginning an exercise programme should consult their physicians to determine the appropriateness of the regime they wish to undertake.

Sex steroids

As we have discussed, overian failure is one of the most significant factors influencing bone loss in young women. Rigidly controlled studies have now shown that oestrogen therapy for the oophorectomised or postmenopausal woman significantly retards bone loss for at least as long as the treatment is provided (Aitken et al, 1973; Lindsay et al, 1976; Recker, Heaney & Saville, 1977; Horsman et al, 1977; Lindsay et al, 1980). In our long-term study, we demonstrated that mestranol (average daily dose 24.8 μg) prevented bone loss, whereas a matching placebo failed (Fig. 7.5) After about 10 years of therapy, height loss was evident among some members of the placebo-treated group, whereas no height loss was seen in the oestrogen-treated group. Radiographs confirmed the presence of vertebral deformities in a significant number of the placebo-treated patients, whereas such changes were absent in the oestrogen-treated group (Table 7.3).

The minimum effective dose of oestrogen appears to be about 0.625 mg conjugated equine oestrogens per day (Lindsay, Hart & Clark, 1984). When

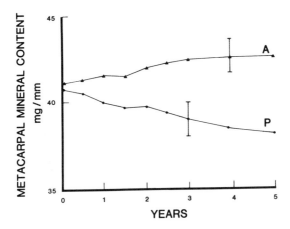

Fig. 7.5 The effect of oestrogen (A) or a placebo (P) on bone mass during a five-year prospective double-blind study in 120 oophorectomised women (from Lindsay et al, 1976, with permission).

Table 7.3 Skeletal changes after ten years of either Oestrogen or Placebo

	Mean height change	Mean weight change	Mean spine score
Oestrogen	− 0.1 cm	− 0.7 kg	0.35
Placebo	− 1.2 cm	+ 3.2 kg	1.65
	$P < 0.05$	$P < 0.01$	$P < 0.005$

*Total spine score for each patient obtained by addition of scores for wedging as one and collapse as two for all thoracic and lumbar vertebrae.

oestrogen therapy is discontinued, bone mass declines at a rate comparable to the immediate postmenopausal period (Lindsay et al, 1978; Horsman et al, 1979). Although the period of therapy required for complete protection is unknown, a significant protective effect might be obtained by periods of therapy in excess of 4–5 years. At least the onset of the high risk period for fracture might be delayed by that period. Weiss et al (1980) have calculated, using retrospective data, at least a 50 per cent reduction in fracture risk with six years of exposure to oestrogen. If this is an overall reduction in all osteoporotic fractures, the expected savings in the USA might be as much as $2 billion per year currently. Moreover, such a reduction in fracture incidence would presumably also reduce the death rate from hip fracture by 50 per cent.

Calculating the cost of provision of such preventive treatment is less easy. Added to the costs of tablet supply and routine care for a relatively large segment of the population must be the possible costs of any complications of therapy, while any added benefits must also be considered. With the prescription of combined or sequential therapy (with an added progestogen) and careful follow-up, the previously described complications of therapy effectively disappear. The incidence of endometrial and breast carcinomata appears to be significantly reduced by therapy (Gambrell et al, 1983). In addition, other possible benefits of continued oestrogen therapy — reduced myocardial incidents (Ross et al, 1981) and longer lifespan — must be taken into account.

Mode of action of oestrogens

There is currently no evidence that oestrogens affect bone directly. Oestrogen receptors have not been found in bone (Chen & Feldman, 1978), and it is generally assumed that oestrogens must function by interaction with the three major hormone systems controlling calcium metabolism: parathyroid hormone, calcitonin, and the vitamin D system. The exact interaction has yet to be elucidated. However, currently, the most acceptable hypothesis for the action of oestrogens assumes that oestrogens stimulate endogenous calcitonin production. Pregnancy has been shown, in some studies, but not all, to stimulate calcitonin levels in women to at least those that occur in the male (Stevenson et al, 1981; Body & Heath, 1983). It has been suggested also that ovulation, when oestrogen levels are highest during the menstrual cycle, is associated with higher calcitonin levels, although this also remains disputed (Pilkin et al, 1978; Barran, 1980). Therapy with oestrogens has been reported to increase plasma calcitonin in women (Stevenson et al, 1981).

Such increments in circulating calcitonin might reduce the flow of calcium from bone to blood, since the only important biological action of calcitonin appears to be osteoclast inhibition and reduction of bone resorption. The subsequent biochemical events which could be postulated in this circumstances, namely a fall in serum calcium, rises in PTH and 1,25 dihydroxyvitamin D, could account for the other known biochemical events which follow oestrogen administration. What data are available, therefore, are in the main consistent with this hypothesis for oestrogen action. However, more detailed studies are still required, and a non-genome-dependent action of oestrogen directly on bone is still a possibility.

Progestogens

Evidence is now accumulating that certain progestogens may also reduce bone loss among postmenopausal women. Urinary calcium excretion is reduced by some progestogens, and progestogens have been shown to protect the oophorectomised rat from bone loss by mechanisms which may be different from those exerted by oestrogens (Lindsay et al, 1978a). In a preliminary study in which we examined the effects of a depot progestogen, we showed that bone loss could be prevented by a progestogen as well as oestrogen (Lindsay et al, 1978b). More recently we have completed a study of two oral 19-nor steroids regularly used as progestogenic compounds. In this study, norethisterone retarded bone loss, while norgestrel was ineffective, in the dose used.

Combined therapy using oestrogen–progestogen combinations is now the treatment of choice for intact postmenopausal women, and perhaps also for oophorectomised women (Gambrell et al, 1983). Combination therapy appears to be as effective as the oestrogen alone in preventing postmenopausal bone loss and also in treatment of the established disease, and there does not appear to be either an additive or synergistic effect on bone mass when a progestogen is added to oestrogen treatment.

Other factors

Clearly the three most important factors influencing the development of postmenopausal osteoporosis are dietary calcium, exercise and gonadal steroids. They are also the ones which can be most readily approached in developing a programme of effective preventive therapy. However, of the other factors which are correctable, advice about cigarette consumption and alcohol abuse is mandatory, for good health reasons as well as specifically for prevention of osteoporosis. The health professional must, of course, be well aware of the low level of success in convincing individuals to reduce or eliminate these habits, and should have available *all* arguments in favor of eradicating such excesses.

Somewhat similarly, reduction in caffeine intake is advisable but often difficult to achieve. Excessive intake of phosphate and animal protein should probably also be avoided, as should overindulgence in calories. Yet, again, these are essentially measures in good health maintenance from which a major spin-off may be reduction of risk of osteoporosis. The essence of preventive medicine remains an active lifestyle and a well-balanced diet.

Additionally, one important approach to the prevention of osteoporosis lies within the physician's scope. Restriction of the therapeutic use of corticosteroids only to those problem cases in which their use becomes vitally necessary, and provision of short-term therapy when possible, would significantly assist preventive steps for osteoporosis. When the primary diagnosis for which such steroid therapy is often symptomatically compelling, the production of steroid osteoporosis, often more rapidly and with greater severity than the physician can predict (especially in an immobile, arthritic, postmenopausal woman) will cause lifelong misery, and the physician must be aware of this. It has been suggested that the use of vitamin D and calcium supplements from the onset of steroid therapy will reduce the incidence and severity of osteoporosis (Hahn, 1978), but this still requires to be confirmed.

The role of vitamins in osteoporosis is controversial, particularly vitamin D. Levels of the active metabolite of vitamin D, 1,25 dihydroxyvitamin D, decrease with age (Gallagher et al, 1979), and may be reduced in a significant proportion of elderly fracture-prone individuals. However, there is no evidence that vitamin D deficiency influences bone loss in younger women, and the use of 1,25 dihydroxyvitamin D is ineffective in reducing bone loss (Christiansen et al, 1981). Since young individuals probably synthesise sufficient vitamin D in skin under most circumstances, we feel that at present there is no place for dietary supplementation using vitamin D. Among older individuals, however, the situation may be different, and further investigation of the requirements for vitamin D in this age group is required.

Osteoporosis in men

While osteoporosis is primarily a disorder of postmenopausal women, a clinically similar syndrome does occur in elderly men, although the frequency of the disorder is significantly lower than among women of comparable ages. In a recent assessment of the risk factors associated with osteoporosis among men (Seeman et al, 1983), one-third had a significant disorder known to affect bone and mineral metabolism, one-half of these receiving long-term glucocorticoid therapy. Use of tobacco and alcohol was also greater in the patients with osteoporosis. Obesity was a protective factor, as is true among women. Hypogonadism was significantly associated with osteoporosis, as in the female. Dietary and exercise patterns were not assessed in this study, but we have no reason to believe that the occurrence of those risk factors would be any different among men than among women.

Preventive advice and therapy for men is, therefore, somewhat similar to that provided for women. Correction of underlying disease, reduction in the abuse of alcohol and tobacco are clearly the most important. Obtaining an adequate calcium intake and continuing exercise throughout life are also recommended. We have found that alocohol abuse is the single most common factor present among young men who present with osteoporosis.

SUMMARY

It is now possible to categorise those individuals who may be at risk from osteoporosis. It may be useful to use the menopause as the time to determine those most at risk and to institute preventive measures at that point, although advice on prevention at a significantly earlier age must not be disregarded.

The risk factors most readily corrected are those of poor diet and lifestyle. Increasing calcium intake, reducing alcohol, caffeine and protein intake may help prevent bone loss. Increasing physical activity may also have beneficial effects, as may reduction or cessation of cigarette use. The potential benefits in general health may be greater than those obtained by any prevention of bone loss, since we cannot as yet determine the effectiveness in terms of fracture prevention of such programmes.

Undoubtedly, the most effective method of preventing bone loss and subsequent fracture is the prescription of oestrogen therapy in combination with a progestogen. Case-control studies suggest that a 50 per cent reduction in fracture risk may be obtained with six years' exposure to oestrogen. Here other potential risks and benefits must be taken into account. Each patient must be reviewed on an individual basis. Therapy and its many implications should be described to the patient before committing the patient and the physician to a relatively prolonged period of treatment requiring careful follow-up. Where bone mass measurements are available, these should be obained prior to treatment and during the treatment period, using the results to assist in determining the need for treatment and the efficacy of the regime provided.

REFERENCES

Aitken J M, Hart D M, Lindsay R 1973 Oestrogen replacement therapy for prevention of osteoporosis after oophorectomy. British Medical Journal 3: 515–518
Albright F, Bloomberg E, Smith P H 1940 Postmenopausal osteoporosis. Transactions of the Association of American Physicians 55: 298–305
Aloia J F, Cohn S H, Ostuni J A, Cane R, Ellis K 1978 Prevention of involutional bone loss by exercise. Annals of Internal Medicine 89: 356–358
Aloia J F, Cohn S H, Babu T, Abesamis C, Kalici N, Ellis K 1978 Skeletal mass and body composition in marathon runners. Metabolism 27: 1793–1796
Barran D T, Whyte M P, Haussler M R, Deftos L J, Slalopotsky E, Avioli L V 1980 Effect of the menstrual cycle on calcium in regulating hormones. Journal of Clinical Endocrinology and Metabolism 50: 377–379
Body J J, Heath H III 1983 Estimates of circulating monomeric calcitonin: physiological studies in normal and thyroidectomized man. Journal of Clinical Endocrinology and Metabolism 57: 897–903
Cann C E, Genant H K, Ettinger B, Gordan G S 1980 Spinal mineral loss in oophorectomized women. Determination by quantitative computed tomography. Journal of the American Medical Association 244: 2056–2059
Chen T L, Feldman D 1978 Distinction between α-fetoprotein and intracellular estrogen receptors: evidence against presence of estradiol receptors in rat bone. Endocrinology 102: 236–244
Christiansen C, Christensen M S, Redbro P, Hagen C, Transbol I 1981 Effect of 1,25 dihydroxyvitamin D_3 in itself or combined with hormone treatment in preventing postmenopausal osteoporosis. European Journal of Clinical Investigation 11: 305–309
Christiansen C, Christensen M S, McNair P, Hagen C, Stocklund K S, Transbol I 1980 Prevention of early postmenopausal bone loss: controlled 2-year study in 315 normal females. European Journal of Clinical Investigation 10:273–279
Daniell H W 1976 Osteoporosis and the slender smoker. Archives of Internal Medicine 136: 298–304
Dequeker J V, Johnston C C 1981 Non-invasive bone measurements. IRL Press, Oxford
Fenton-Lewis A 1981 Fracture of neck of the femur; changing incidence. British Medical Journal 283: 1217–1220
Fogelman I, Bessent R G, Cohen H N, Hart D M, Lindsay R 1980 Skeletal uptake of diphosphonate: method for prediction of postmenopausal osteoporosis. Lancet ii: 667–670
Gallagher J C, Melton L J, Riggs B L, Bergstrath E 1980 Epidemiology of fractures of the proximal femur in Rochester, Minnesota. Clinical Orthopedics 150: 168–171
Gallagher JC, Riggs B L, Eisman J, Hamstra A, Arnaud S B, Deluca H F 1979 Intestinal calcium absorption and serum vitamin D metabolites in normal subjects and osteopenic patients. Journal of Clinical Investigation 64: 729–736
Gambrell R D, Bagnell C A, Greenblatt R B 1983 Role of estrogens and progesterone in the etiology and prevention of endometrial cancer: review. American Journal of Obstetrics and Gynecology 146: 696–707
Garn S M 1970 The earlier gain and later loss of cortical bone. Thomas, Springfield
Genant H K, Cann C E 1983 Clinical impact of quantitative computed tomography for vertebral mineral assessment. In: Margulis A R, Gooding C A (eds) Diagnostic radiology: 26th postgraduate course. University of California Printing Office, University of California, San Francisco, p 445-448

Gordan G, Vaughan C 1976 Clinical management of the osteoporoses. Publishing Sciences Group, Acton, Mass.
Hahn T J 1978 Corticosteroid induced osteoporosis. Archives of Internal Medicine 138: 882–885
Heaney R P 1965 A unified concept of osteoporosis. American Journal of Medicine 39: 377–880
Heaney R P, Recker R R, Saville P D 1977 Calcium balance and calcium requirements in middle-aged women. American Journal of Clinical Nutrition 30: 1603–1611
Heaney R P, Recker R R, Saville P D 1978a Menopausal changes in bone remodelling. Journal of Laboratory and Clinical Medicine 92: 964–970
Heaney R P, Recker R R, Saville P D 1978b Menopausal changes in calcium balance performance. Journal of Laboratory and Clinical Medicine 92: 953–963
Horsman A, Nordin B E C, Crilly R G 1979 Effect on bone of withdrawal of oestrogen therapy. Lancet ii: 33
Horsman A, Gallagher J C, Simpson M, Nordin B E C 1977 Prospective trial of oestrogen and calcium in postmenopausal women. British Medical Journal 2: 789–792
Hui S L, Wiske P S, Norton J A, Johnston C C, Jr 1982 A prospective study of change in bone mass with age in postmenopausal women. Journal of Chronic Diseases 35: 715–725
Jensen J S, Tondevold E 1979 Mortality after hip fractures. Acta Orthopaedica Scandinavica 50: 161–167
Krolner B, Toft B, Nielsen S P, Tondevold E 1983 Physical exercise as prophylaxis against involutional bone loss: a controlled trial. Clinical Science 64: 541–546
Lindsay R, Hart D M, Aitken J M, MacDonald E B, Anderson J B, Clark A 1976 Long-term prevention of postmenopausal osteoporosis by oestrogen. Lancet i: 1038–1041
Lindsay R, Hart D M, MacLean A, Clark A C, Kraszewski A, Garwood J 1978 Bone response to termination of oestrogen treatment. Lancet i: 1325–1327
Lindsay R, Hart D M, Forrest C, Baird C 1980 Prevention of Spinal osteoporosis in oophorectomized women. Lancet ii: 1151–1154
Lindsay R 1981 The influence of cigarette smoking on bone mass and bone loss. In: DeLuca H F, Frost H M, Jee W S S, Johnston C C, Jr, Parfitt A M (eds) Osteoporosis: recent advances in pathogenesis and treatment. University Park Press, Baltimore, p 477
Lindsay R, Herrington B S 1983 Osteoporotic fractures in the United States of America. Seminars in Reproductive Endocrinology 1: 55–67
Lindsay R, Hart D M, Clark D M 1984 The minimum effective dose of estrogen for prevention of postmenopausal bone loss. Obstetrics and Gynecology 63: 759–763
Lindsay R, Hart D M, Aitken J M, Purdie D 1978a The effect of ovarian sex steroids on bone mineral status in the oophorectomized rat and in the human. Postgraduate Medical Journal 54 (S. 2): 50–58
Lindsay R, Hart D M, Purdie D, Ferguson M M, Clark A S, Kraszewski A 1978b Comparative effects of oestrogen and a progestogen on bone loss in postmenopausal women. Clinical Science and Molecular Medicine 54: 193–195
Matkovic V, Kostial K, Simonovic I, Buzina R, Brodarec A, Nordin B E 1979 Bone status and fracture rates in two regions of Yugoslavia. American Journal of Clinical Nutrition 32: 540–549
Mazess R B 1979 Non-invasive measurement of bone. In: Barzel U (ed) Osteoporosis II. Grune & Stratton, New York, p 5–26
Montoye H J, Smith E L, Fardon D F, Howley E T 1980 Bone mineral in senior tennis players. Scandanavian Journal Sports Science 2: 26–32
Pilkin R M, Reynolds W A, Williams G A, Hargil G K 1978 Calcium regulating hormones during the menstrual cycle. Journal of Clinical Endocrinology and Metabolism 47: 626–632
Recker R R, Saville S D, Heaney R P 1977 Effect of estrogens and calcium carbonate on bone loss in postmenopausal women. Annals of Internal Medicine 87: 649–655
Riggs B L, Wahner H W, Dunn W L, Mazess R B, Oxford K P, Melton L J III 1981 Differential changes in bone mineral density of the appendicular and axial skeleton with aging: relationship to spinal osteoporosis. Journal of Clinical Investigation 67: 328–355
Ross R K, Paganini-Hill A, Mack T M, Arthur M, Henderson B E 1981 Menopausal estrogen therapy and protection from death from ischemic heart disease. Lancet 1: 858–860
Saville P D 1965 Changes in bone mass with age and alcoholism. Journal of Bone and Joint Surgery (Am) 47: 492–499
Saville P D 1970 Observations on 80 women with osteoporotic spine fractures. In: Barzel U (ed) Osteoporosis. Grune & Stratton, New York, p 38–46

Seeman E, Malton L J III, O'Fallon W M, Riggs B L 1983 Risk factors for spinal osteoporosis in men. American Journal of Medicine 75: 977–983

Smith E L, Reddan W Smith P E 1981 Physical activity and calcium modalities for bone mineral increase in aged women. Medicine and Science in Sports and Exercise 13: 60–64

Stevenson J C, Abeyasekerg G L, Hillyard C J, Phang K G, MacIntyre I 1981 Calcitonin and the calcium regulating hormones in postmenopausal women: effect of oestrogens. Lancet i: 693–695

Wallace W A 1983 The increasing incidence of fractures of the proixmal femur: an orthopaedic epidemic. Lancet i: 1413–1414

Weiss N S, Dr P H, Ure C L, Ballard J H, Williams A R, Daling J R 1980 Decreased risk of fractures of the hip and lower forearm with postmenopausal use of estrogen. New England Journal of Medicine 303: 1195–1198

8
Sandra L. Baker

The preventability of falls

INTRODUCTION

In the course of evolution from the quadripedal to the bipedal gait, human beings have become increasingly liable to fall, and particularly so during old age. The majority of falls suffered by old people occasion no actual physical harm, but the fear engendered may be a potent cause of increasing immobility and ultimately of loss of independent existence in the community. The desirability of prevention of falls is therefore evident, both on humanitarian and economic grounds. In order to consider prevention it is fundamental to define the extent and causes of the problem to determine factors which may be subject to modification.

If balance is considered to be 'a set of strategies which maintain the body upright by correcting the forces of displacement', then a fall may be defined as 'an involuntary displacement of the body resulting in the subject finding himself on the ground'. These definitions will be borne in mind in the ensuing discussion.

THE EPIDEMIOLOGY OF FALLS

Any study on the subject of fall incidence in the elderly must be critically evaluated. The majority of papers on the subject have been retrospective rather than prospective, with the inherent problem of errors of recall by the subject. This problem is amplified in the confused elderly, where eyewitness accounts may prove more accurate. Many falls do not cause physical injury, making injury-reporting a serious underestimate of fall frequency. It has been estimated that over three million falls in those aged 65 and over occur per annum, less than 1 per cent of which result in proximal femoral fracture. Finally, fall incidence differs with the population as to whether they are at home or within an institutional setting.

One of the earliest studies to draw attention to the problem of falls in an elderly population at home was that of Sheldon (1948). A random sample of 400 people aged 65 and over in Wolverhampton were visited and a comprehensive questionnaire on health, including falls, was completed. Some 43 per cent of females and 21 per cent of males were reported as having fallen or 'shown a tendency to fall', though the period of time involved was not defined. He showed a linear increase in 'liability to fall' with age, with a more marked tendency in females than in males.

Exton-Smith (1977) looked at 963 individuals (427 females and 536 males) who took part in a nutritional survey in London. His figures were similar to those of Sheldon (1948), showing an increasing tendency to fall with advancing age, especially in females, with an apparent slight reduction in tendency to fall in men aged over 85. This reduction could be explained by the small numbers of men involved or may represent a survivor population of the extremely fit elderly. Whereas Sheldon suggested that the likelihood of falling starts at approximately 60 years of age in both sexes, it is possible that this tendency starts as early as 45 to 50 years of age.

Wild et al (1981) in a prospective study of 125 people who fell at home interviewed the individuals again at three and twelve months after the fall for evidence of further falls. These falls were compared to the numbers spontaneously reported by these subjects to their general practitioners. The interviewed group recalled almost twenty times as many falls as those reported to the general practitioner, again highlighting difficulties in obtaining accurate figures. The interviewed group, although probably still representing an underestimate of the true figures, shows an estimated incidence in the 65–74 age group of 140 per 1000 per annum, which rises with age (Table 8.1).

Turning to accidents within the home, it is found that falls are by far the most common type of accident (Leake 1964; Gray, 1966). On informatiion obtained from death certification it was found that between 80 and 90 per cent of fatal home accidents in the eldery result directly from falls. Gray (1966) in her report to the Royal Society for the Prevention of Accidents compared people who had had home accidents in a twelve-month period with an age/sex matched control group. The social characteristics of the two groups were compared, but no comment made on their medical condition. Further study of the circumstances of the fall within the home and the

Table 8.1 Estimated incidence of falls (Wild et al, 1980)

Age/sex group	Estimated annual falls reported	Incidence per 1000: falls recalled at 12 months
Males 65–74	4	140
75–84	114	400
85 and over	18	333
Females 65–74	5	667
75–84	33	425
85 and over	60	967

These figures suggest that, on average, each person aged 75 and over will fall each year.

medical condition of the faller is needed to assess relevant environmental and fall characteristics.

People staying in hospital or living in residential accommodation are more likely to fall than those living in their own homes, mainly because the former group are 'les well'. As the environment of the hospital or residential home is more accessible to controlled assessment, figures for incidence and prevalence of falls are more likely to be accurate in these settings.

Falls are frequently the reason for admission to a geriatric unit, and papers such as that of Naylor & Rosen (1970) suggest that approximately one quarter of admissions are directly caused by falls. Most of these patients were suffering from a significant physical illness, and they suggested that falls were a symptom of this underlying disorder.

Falls occurring whilst the old person is in hospital have also been studied (Fine, 1959). Morris 8 Isaacs (1980) found an incidence of falling of 422 per thousand per annum in their sample. As with people at home, the likelihood of falling increased with age up to 85 years, and declined slightly thereafter. Three-quarters of those who fell sustained no physical injury, whilst 2 per cent of the falls resulted in proximal femoral fracture.

In England and Wales over 100 000 elderly people live in residential accommodation, and Morfitt (1979), looking at residents treated at a hospital accident and emergency department, found 98 per cent of injuries were due to falls. Both accident and fracture rates were significantly higher than for an age/sex matched population living in their own or their relatives' homes. Similarly, a Canadian study of elderly people in residential accommodation (Gryfe et al, 1977) gave an incidence of falls of 668 per 1000 per annum. Eighty per cent of those falls caused no injury, whilst 6 per cent resulted in fractures, of which 1 per cent were proximal femoral fractures.

It would appear that there is an absolute increase in the number of falls resulting in fracture of the femur. A study by Lewis (1981) considering secular trends in femoral fracture showed that in London in a ten-year period the number of admissions to hospital for this condition had increased by 55 per cent for men and 65 per cent for women. The overall bed occupancy increase was of the order of 48 per cent, even though the average duration of stay in females fell from 43 to 39 days over this same period. No conclusions were drawn as to whether this increase represented a true increase in the number of falls over the decade, or whether the proportion of falls resulting in femoral fracture had risen. It can be seen that falls are a common occurrence, causing much morbidity and a significant mortality.

In spite of the considerable variation in incidence and prevalence figures, depending on the method of study, an age-related trend of increasing risk of falling with advancing age is common to all. Further information of value in determining preventability of falling can be obtained by looking at the fall and the person who has fallen in each age band.

CLASSIFICATION OF FALLS AND FALLERS

The literature on classification by cause of fall is confusing, often combining a mixture of pathological and purely descriptive terms as a frame of reference. Of necessity most classifications of cause of fall rely on the recall of the event by the faller, often at a time long after the reference fall. Not only are these statements open to errors of recall, but also to 'errors of nationalisation'. The statement 'I must have tripped (slipped)' may well represent an attempt on the part of the old person to explain a fall for which the cause is uncertain. In spite of these inherent difficulties, classification of falls and fallers is of value in deciding prognosis and possible methods of intervention to prevent recurrence.

The faller

A broad classification based on frequency of falls is useful in defining general characteristics of fallers as follows:
1. *Occasional falls* — gait and balance are normal and general health is good.
2. *Intermittent or intercurrent fallers* — subject to intermittent disturbances of function, but gait and balance normal between falls. The intermittant dysfunction may be caused by an acute illness or transient disorder of the circulatory system.
3. *Recurrent fallers* — in whom gait and balance are persistently abnormal and whose general health is poor.

The prognosis both in terms of independent survival and with regard to further falls diminishes from group 1 to group 3. The characteristics of the recurrent faller will be considered in further detail after a consideration of factors involved in the individual fall.

The fall

In describing an individual fall an attempt is usually made to distinguish between 'accidental' falls, in which an external hazard is thought to be responsible, and 'non-accidental' falls. External hazards include wet or slippery floors, trailing wires, edges of carpets and objects inappropriately placed on the floor. 'Non-accidental' falls are those in which the prime cause is thought to be within the individual, the environment playing only a minor role. The dichotomy is far from absolute, and it is probably better to consider the difference as quantitative rather than qualitative. The trip which would be easily righted in a young person may lead to a fall in an older individual whose corrective mechanisms are less capable of correcting sudden displacements.

Accidental falls, usually described by the person as a trip of a slip, are a common cause of falls in the elderly. Several studies have suggested that between a third and a half of all falls in the home are accidental falls (Sheldon, 1963; Lucht, 1971; Prudham et al, 1979), while other studies (Wild et al, 1981) have suggested that fewer than 10 per cent can be directly attributed to external hazards. The differences are not easily understood, though there is concurence in studies that the proportion of falls due to environmental factors because less common with increasing age.

Useful insight as to possible external hazards may be obtained by looking at when and where the fall occurred, and in what activity the individual was engaged at the time of the fall.

Time of the fall

In the home 85 per cent of falls occur during the day (Lucht, 1971), with the highest incidence in the mid-morning, mid-afternoon and late evening. In residential accommodation Rodstein (1964) found the highest incidence in the morning and between 5.00 and 9.00 p.m., whilst hospital studies e.g. that of Fine (1959) show mid-morning 2.00–3.00 p.m. and 1.00–2.00 a.m. as 'peak periods' for falls. Here, factors other than the person's activity at the time of falling played a significant part. The highest incidence of falls corresponded with lowest staffing levels, stressing the need for well-positioned nursing stations in situations where a few nurses have large numbers of patients to care for. The period between 1.00 and 2.00 a.m. is a time when old people may be visiting the toilet, at a time when lighting levels are reduced.

As well as diurnal variation, seasonal variation in the incidence of certain types of fall has been demonstrated. Outdoor falls causing fracture of the femoral neck occur most commonly during July and August (Brocklehurst et al, 1976), whilst indoor falls causing fractures peak during March and April. Brocklehurst's (1976) results, however, show only trends, and do not reach statistical significance. Other studies e.g. that of Prudham, Grimley Evans and Wandless (1979) have failed to show a seasonal variation in fractures of the femoral neck.

Site of the fall

Indoor falls usually occur in the living room or bedroom, where the person spends most of his or her time. Outdoor falls are commonly on the front or back steps of the house, or on the pavement nearby. The stairs within the home have been cited as a potential hazard; Sheldon (1963) showed in his group that one-third of falls occurred in this site. He considered that the first or last few steps are the most hazardous, with falls whilst ascending being more dangerous than falls whilst descending. Other groups e.g. Gray (1966) and Lucht (1971) have reported a lower incidence of falls in the vicinity of the stairs, but still view stairs as potentially dangerous, particularly in older homes with steep ill-lit staircases. The provision of two handrails with a cue on the rail to warn when the person is approaching the last step may be all that is needed to reduce risks. In other cases, life on the ground floor with the necessary furniture and toilet rearrangements may have to be considered.

Most falls outside of hospital or residential accommodation are associated with everyday activities such as walking, doing the housework or gardening. Injudicious activities, e.g. hanging curtains whilst standing on a chair, are distinctly uncommon as causes, but should clearly be advised against.

Within the hospital setting most falls occur within the vicinity of the bed, and are associated with getting into or out of bed, or toileting. Falls from chair or wheelchair usually occur when the person is standing up or sitting down, but slipping out of the chair once seated is uncommon. The correct size of chair or wheelchair will reduce the incidence of falls on standing or sitting.

The physiological and pathological conditions within the faller which increase the tendency to fall will now be considered.

The faller

Sway and balance

The random movements of an individual about a fixed point when standing with the feet comfortably apart (sway) were first noticed by Hinsdale (1887). The relationship, however, between an increase in sway (representing a decrease in postural stability) and the likelihood of falling in old age has only been studied in recent years. One does not have to search far to discover the reason for this, considering the complexity of both the physiology and measurement of sway and balance. A working knowledge of the mechanisms involved in maintaining the erect posture is desirable, as a failure of this control may cause falls.

Physiology of sway

The centre of mass of the human body lies somewhere in the region of the second sacral vertebra. Any movement of the individual will cause the centre of mass to move away from a position over the centre of the support base provided by the feet to a potentially unstable position. Body displacement must be kept under vigilant surveillance of the nervous system and its righting reactions, or overbalancing may occur.

The neurophysiology of postural control is complex. The three major afferent components of balance are proprioception (mainly joint mechanoreceptors), the vestibular labyrinth and vision, with an interdependence of these modalities in normal individuals. Central processing occurs in the brain and spinal cord, and the control of balance is effected by the efferent pool of cranial and spinal motoneurones.

Vestibular mechanisms

The vestibular component of postural control declines with ascent of the evolutionary scale. In humans the vestibular labyrinth, consisting of the semicircular canals and the otolith organ (the saccule and utricle) may help in the maintenance of the head in the erect position. The semicircular canals signal acceleration reflexes, whilst the saccule and utricle sense positional reflexes. Humans are not wholly dependent upon vestibular mechanisms under conditions of normal static posture, but these may become of greater importance when the support base is unstable, as in walking over uneven ground or when underwater (Purdon-Martin, 1967). With intact proprioceptive and visual mechanisms, normal balance may be found when vestibular function is completely lost, if stresses are not applied. If, however, subjects with vestibular dysfunction are subject to rapid tilting, they are more likely to fall than those with intact vestibular systems. Vestibular function is known to decline with age, but as it usually only serves as a 'back-up' system when proprioceptive or visual input is defective, its role in the genesis of falls is uncertain.

Visual mechanisms

In common with vestibular mechanisms, visual input appears not to be critical in the maintenance of static balance. When vision conflicts with other information, balance in adults can be maintained by reliance on proprioceptive input alone (Coady & Nelson, 1978). Conflicting evidence from Witkin & Warpner (1950) suggests that some females place a greater reliance on vision than an proprioceptive information, but their findings have not been confirmed by other groups. In the elderly, a relatively greater reliance on vision has been suggested by Over (1966), with falls resulting from conflict between visual, proprioceptive and vestibular inputs. As visual disorder is so common in the elderly, this facet should be minimised by regular refraction and ophthalmological intervention, as indicated.

Proprioceptive mechanisms

The apophyseal joints of the cervical spine have mechanoreceptors which are of important in stabilising posture and gait (Wyke, 1979). These mechanoreceptors relay in adjacent segments of the spinal cord and project to the medial longitudinal fasciculus and cerebellum. Other fibres relay via the thalamus to the parietal and paracentral regions of the cerebral cortex to serve kinaesthetic and postural sensibility. Cervical apophyseal mechanoreceptor dysfunction leads to nytagmus, ataxia, vertigo and arm dyspraxia, and may closely resemble vertebrobasilar ischaemia. The provision of a cervical collar to a patient who is presumed, incorrectly, to have vertebrobasilar ischaemia due to cervical spondylosis may have increase in his or her instability by a further reduction in mechanoreceptor input.

The mechanisms mentioned, usually combined with osteoarthrosis of hips and knees, combine to cause an increase in sway in old age and a gait characterised by slower speed, shorter step length, and a longer double support time (the time spent with both feet on the ground during walking).

Postural stability can be quantified by measuring the movement of the centre of foot pressure which represents the body's response to movement of the centre of mass, or directly from body sway. In measurements of these two parameters, sway is the easier one to study.

Sheldon (1963) looked at sway in 268 subjects aged 6–96 using a triangular aluminium frame from which projected a pointer with a pencil writing on a sheet of paper. He found that, after a period of 'maturation' in childhood, sway remained at a minimum throughout adult life, until, at about 60, sway began to increase with advancing age. The general impression was that falls were more likely in those with increased sway.

Overstall et al (1977), considering the relationship between falls and sway in the elderly, compared 243 subjects aged 60–96 with 63 hospial workers aged 18–59. Sway measurements were made with Wright's ataxiamter (Wright, 1971) consisting of a box on the floor from which projects a vertical mast attached by a thread to a belt worn around the subject's waist. Movement is communicated via a double ratchet mechanism to a calibrated dial, each unit represent $3\frac{1}{3}°$ of sway. Sway is measured as the total angular movement in the anteroposterior plane only, summated irrespective of sign. A fall history was obtained from their subjects, who were then divided into three groups; those who had not fallen, those who had fallen only as a result of tripping, and those with 'postural falls' (defined as being due to giddiness drop attacks, head turning, loss of balance, or whilst rising from bed or chair). They found that sway was greater in females than in males at all ages (see also Hasselkus & Shambes, 1975), and that sway increased in both sexes with age. No difference in amplitude of sway was found between those who had fallen as a result of tripping and those who had no falls. Sway was significantly increased in females who had fallen due to 'postural causes', and in men whose falls were attributed to a 'loss of balance'.

Fernie et al (1982) reported results which are at variance with the above study. In a double-blind study of the relationship between sway and fall frequency in the institutionalised elderly, they could demonstrate no sex-related difference in mean speed of sway nor any age-related increase in the amplitude of sway. Mean speed of sway was found to be greater for those who had fallen one or more times in a year than those who had not fallen, and the group as a whole swayed more than people living in their own homes. Group trends could be demonstrated, but prediction as to any one individuals's risk of falling could not be made.

The differing results may be explained by the different study populations, and as to whether sway is measured as total angular sway or sway in the anteropsterior plane only. Further study is needed to determine which populations would benefit from formal gait analysis and which measurement is most appropriate. Clinical tests of gait and balance however, need not be elaborate, and much can be learnt be observing the subject walk, rise from a chair, and perform Romberg's test. A further simple test involves the response to a light tap on the sternum, a displacement rapidly corrected by those with normal balance, but inadequately by those whose balance is poor.

The management of individuals who have demonstrable abnormalities of balance and gait should be to eliminate environmental hazards wherever possible, increase illumination and provide additional support, e.g. grab rails in a situation where instability is likely.

Cardiac and haemodynamic risk factors

Impairment of cardiac output, leading to cerebral hypoperfusion may cause 'dizziness' if short, or unconsciousness with falls is prolonged. Cardiac syncope (defined as a reversible loss of conciousness secondary to cerebral ischaemia) may be related to reduced cerebral blood flow or an alteration in blood constituents.

A vasovagal attack ('a faint') is due to a vagally mediated bradyardia and profound dilation of veins in the gut and skeletal muscles. Episodes usually occur when the individual rises from the sitting or lying position, and frequently in overheated environments. The attack may be precipitated by intense emotional response such as fear or disgust, and is usually accompanied by a prodromal disequilibrium, sweating, pallor and nausea. The individual falls to the ground and lies motionless for several seconds, after which consciousness is rapidly regained. If he or she is not allowed to lie flat, cerebral anoxia may be prolonged, leading to convulsions and delayed return of consciousness. The vasovagal attack is not indicative of any serious underlying pathology in most cases, but increases in old people taking drugs which may reduce blood volume, in whom attacks may coexist with postural hypotension.

Postural (orthostatic) hypotension. Postural hypotension is defined as a fall in systolic blood pressure greater than 20 mmHg on standing from the lying (or sitting) position. In normal individuals, baroreceptors present in the carotid body, aortic arch and elsewhere respond to arterial hypotension by causing a sympathetically-mediated increase in blood pressure and reflex tachycardia. In postural hypotension these mechanisms fail to occur, causing blood to pool in the capacitance vessels of the legs and gut on standing. Cardiac output and blood pressure are reduced, the brain is inadequately perfused and consciousness may be lost. Because the hypotension develops so rapidly, the fall is often not preceded by pallor, sweating, etc. as occurs in a vasovagal attack.

Defects in the baroreceptor response may occur in afferent or efferent sides of the reflex arc, or in its central connections. There may not be a total failure of the system in all cases, as some individuals are able to maintain blood pressure in the face of impaired baroreceptor response by a rise in the plasma renin levels. If diuretic or other treatment is instilled, the precarious homoeostasis rapidly decompensates, leading to postural hypotension.

Between 8 and 24 per cent of ambulant people aged 65 and over have postural hypotension as defined above, and the majority are asymptomatic. Postural hypotension is more likely to cause falls in those people who also have other risk factors, e.g. poor mobility or increased sway.

Postural hypotension is most commonly not associated with other nervous system abnormalities ('idiopathic' postural hypotension as described by Bradbury & Eggleston, 1925).

Other causes of postural hypotension include the following:
1. Parkinson's disease — may be due to the disease itself or L-dopa treatment
2. Peripheral neuropathy e.g. diabetes, alcoholism
3. Cerebrovascular disease
4. Sodium deficiency } may be diuretic-induced
5. Potassium deficiency
6. Drugs with hypotensive action: antihypertensives, diuretics, phenothiazines, benzodiazepines, antidepressants (may also cause cardiac arrhythmias) and alcohol.
7. The Shy-Drager syndrome consisting of a failue of the automic (particularly the sympathetic) nervous system. Additional features include Parkinsonism, urinary difficulties, lack of sweating and impotence.

Management of falls due to postural hypotension should be aimed at the cause. Drugs which have hypotensive action should be removed, with substitution, if necessary, of a more suitable drug. L-dopa preparations should always be combined with a dopa-decarboxylase inhibitor (either carbidopa or benserazide) to prevent peripheral breakdown, as these breakdown products have hypotensive action. Electrolyte disturbances, if present, should be promptly connected but as the majority of these electrolyte disturbances will be diuretic-induced, the clinician must ask himself whether a diuretic is really necessary. Conditions such as postural oedema are more likely to be due to venous insufficiency than cardiac failure, so diuretics may be inappropriate.

If no secondary cause is found, or correction of the underlying cause is not possible, a variety of antigravity supports to ameliorate the condition are available. Elastic stockings rarely prove to be sufficient, but light bandaging, worn day and night, may prove effective in compressing capacitance vessels in the legs. Advice should be given on methods of avoiding rapid postural change, e.g. sitting up in bed and letting the legs hang for thirty seconds before standing.

A variety of drugs are effective in preventing postural hypotension but some, e.g. phenylephrine, have only a transitory effect, whilst others, e.g. tyramine plus tranyclypromine, are effective but can cause sudden severe hypertension. Hydrocortisone 0.1 mg to 1 mg daily is usually effective, but potassium supplementation is needed to combat hypokalaemia. It has recently been suggested that endogenous prostaglandins may act as ß-blockers on peripheral vasculature, inducing hypotension in the isolated (idiopathic) variety. Inhibition of prostaglandin synthesis by indomethacin 25–50 mg three times daily has been successful in some instances. In all cases where drug treatment is used for the condition, the blood pressure and serum electrolyte concentrations must be closely monitored.

Carotid sinus hypersensitivity. Carotid sinus hypersensitivity as a cause of falling is undoubtedly over-diagnosed, but is amenable to treatment if it should prove to be the cause. As previously described, the carotid body baroreceptor, situated at the junction of internal and external carotid arteries, responds to an increase in blood pressure by causing a vagally-mediated bradycardia and hypotension. On head-turning in certain cases (particularly if a tight collar is worn), extreme bradycardia and/or hypotension can occur, with loss of consciousness. This diagnosis can only be substantiated when, upon carotid sinus massage, a significant blood pressure drop or e.c.g. demonstrable bradycardia can be shown.

Insertion of a permanent demand pacemaker will correct some cases, though, when extreme bradycardia and hypotension occur, bilateral carotid sinus denervation may prove necessary.

Cardiac Dysfunction. Structural lesions, e.g. aortic stenosis or mitral valve prolapse, may lead to loss of consciousness and falls, and are surgically correctable in some instances. Cardiac dysrhythmias, particularly episodic heart block, may certainly cause loss of consciousness, but again their significance has probably been overestimated. The demonstration of a cardiac dysrhythmia on the e.c.g. of a person who suffers falls does not establish cause and effect unless the two clearly occur simultaneously.

Though the literature on the relationship between cardiac dysrhythmias and falls is somewhat confusing, some statements can be made with a reasonable degree of certainty. In the elderly, in contrast to fit young people, transient atrioventricular block, sinus bradycardia etc. must be considered as pathological. The finding of chronic complete heart block, bifascicular block, or the bradyarrhythmic variant of the sick sinus syndrome are indications for pacing, whether falls occur or not. If first-degree heart block or bundle branch block are present on the e.c.g., a clear relationship between falls and arrhythmia is necessary before pacing is considered. Tachy or bradyarrhythmias demonstrated on prolonged ambulatory monitoring should ideally be compared with a patient-kept diary of events to determine their relationship to 'funny turns'. If, after due consideration an arrhythmia is suspected as contributing to falls, the trial of an effective anti-arrhythmic may be justified to assess possible benefits.

Drop attacks. A drop attack is a fall, without warning, after which the sufferer is unable to rise for a variable period of time. Consciousness is not lost during an attack, and there are no neurological sequelae. Sheldon (1960), who attributed 58 of 125 falls to drop attacks, described a loss of motor power in legs and trunk due to sudden loss of tone in antigravity muscles. He found that presure on the soles of the feet could restore this power in some instances, a finding not reproduced by other workers.

Stevens & Mathews (1973) drew attention to the fact that the condition is virtually confined to women, findings similar to that of the 1977 study of Overstall et al (1977). With advancing age, males form a higher proportion of cases, though the female preponderance still remains.

The cause or causes of drop attacks remain obscure and, though there is a definite relationship to vertebrobasilar ischaemia, this cannot be the only explanation, as drop attacks occur in young pregnant females in whom cervical spondylosis or vertebral atheroma are unlikely. Until the mechanisms are better elucidated, prevention is not possible.

Finally, other neurological causes of falls, and their possible management, will be considered.

Giddiness

The complaint of dizziness or giddiness, which individuals usually use to describe a feeling of disequilibrium, increases with advancing age. Some 16 per cent of females and 20 per cent of males aged 75 and over complain of this symptom, compared to approximately 5 per cent of people aged 65–74. As was pointed out by Sheldon (1960), giddiness is only associated with falls in a proportion of cases, as an attack may develop slowly enough for the affected person to grasp a support or sit down.

'Giddiness' as a symptom may relate to vertebrobasilar insufficiency, vestibular dysfunction etc., particularly if precipitated by head-turning. If true vertebrobasilar ischaemia is present, other neurological features are commonly present, e.g. visual disturbance, dysarthria or transient sensory or motor disturbances. Symptoms, including falls, may be lessened by provision of a cervical collar with or without the antiplatelet agents dipyridamole, aspirin or sulphinpyrazone.

Epilepsy

The incidence of idiopathic and symptomatic epilepsies rises with age and can cause falls in some instances. A history of convulsive movement, tongue-biting and incontinence may be available, but more often than not a reliable report or eyewitness account cannot be obtained. Diagnostic problems also exist in that e.e.g.s in the elderly have a higher incidence of non-specific abnormalities which increase with advancing age, making interpretation more difficult. Further tests may be required, e.g. brain scan or computerised axial tomography, if epilepsy secondary to cerebral tumour, subdural haematoma etc. is suspected. The management of secondary epilepsy is indicated by the precipitating cause.

In cases where history and corroborative evidence suggest idiopathic epilepsy as a cause of falls, a trial of anticonvulsants may be warranted.

Normal-pressure hydrocephalus (n.p.h.).

Rarely, falls may be due to normal-pressure hydrocephalus, a syndrome consisting of dementia, abnormal gait and incontinence of urine, described by Hakim & Roberts (1965). The syndrome may occur in cerebrovascular disease or after inflammatory cerebral conditions e.g. meningitis or subarachnoid haemorrhage. There is internal (communicating) hydrocephalus with a normal pressure of the cerebrospinal fluid.

The characteristic fall in n.p.h. occurs whilst standing or walking and is not associated with loss of consciousness.

Diagnosis is suggested by the clinical history, confirmation being obtained by pressure-flow studies of the cerebrospinal fluid and demonstration of ventricular dilation on computerised axial tomography. The insertion of a ventriculo-atrial or similar shunt is the only effective line of treatment in these instances.

As may be seen from the preceding discussion, there are many possible causes of falls, the management of which depends on the precipitating factors. Though some of these causes are not preventible, it is possible to devise a programme aimed at fall prevention, bearing in mind these risk factors.

PREVENTION OF FALLS

In devising a programme intended to prevent (or reduce) falls, the following factors need to be considered:
1. Identifying those at risk before they have fallen (primary prevention)
2. Attending to environmental hazards
3. Medical assessment of fallers with regard to drug treatment and specific remediable conditions
4. Specific measures to improve mobility and agility in fallers
5. Providing aids to summon help in those who have fallen.

Identifying those at risk of falling (primary prevention)

In an ideal world, all people aged 65 and over would be assessed as to their risk of falling, with appropriate preventive action taken. As this is not a realistic task with present health service staffing levels, assessment may be limited to those with the highest risk. Persons at greatest risk of falling are the household elderly who are aged 75 or over. A general practitioner with between 2000 and 2500 on his list will have between 50 and 90 such individuals. Home visiting of this group by himself, a health visitor, or district nurse is feasible in order to identify special risk factors.

Attending to environmental hazards

The correction of potential hazards within the home may be suggested by a health visitor or district nurse during the visit. Aids to mobility, grab rails, raised toilet seats, etc. may also be recommended and ordered at this time to reduce the risks in special situations. Such simple measures as advising increasing lighting may be sufficient to prevent falls occurring when illumination is inadequate.

The elderly population and their relatives should be made aware of the role of the environmental health officer (formerly known as the public health inspector). His part played in dealing with the risks of pollution, infestation, etc. is well known, but his authority in dealing with disrepair of rented houses, improvement grants etc., to modify environmental hazards is often neglected.

Medical assessment

A domiciliary review of the old person's medication may indicate drugs with hypotensive action, which should be withdrawn if possible. The person's health should be assessed and further referral for investigations or second opinion to the hospital considered to correct remediable illness.

Specific measures to improve mobility and agility

Domiciliary or day-hospital physiotherapy may help to improve muscular strength, agility and mobility in the more severely immobile. In those who have previously fallen, methods of getting up again may be taught in the event of recurrence.

Providing aids to summon help

Even after risk factors have been eliminated as far as possible, falls are still likely to occur. Methods of summoning help for the faller, such as telephones, alarms etc., should be provided to those considered to be of high risk of falling again. Though most old people who have fallen summon help by shouting or banging on the wall, provision of a telephone can be nonetheless useful. The failure of a person to answer the telephone to a regular caller may alert that caller to the possibility of the elderly person having fallen or become ill. Similarly regular visiting programmes by neighbours, friends, etc. will help to keep a check on his or her welfare.

Alarm systems deserve a special mention as often they are too few in number and too high to be reached by a person who has fallen. To be effective, regular spacing of alarm buttons at a height accessible to the faller is needed.

THE FUTURE OF FALL PREVENTION PROGRAMMES

As yet the cost-effectiveness, effect and even the feasibility of these, or similar measures, have not been assessed. Clearly, intervention studies and further research on factors causing falls are of urgent importance. With falls having such a profound impact on the old person, both economically and in terms of quality of life, can we afford to neglect the fall or the faller?

REFERENCES

Bradbury S, Eggleston C 1925 American Heart Journal 1: 73–78
Brocklehurst J C, Duncan-Roberston, James-Groom P 1982 Clinical correlates of sway in old age — sensory modalities. Age and Ageing 2: 1–11
Coady K A, Nelson A J 1978 Physical Therapeutics 58: 35–40
Exton-Smith A N 1977 Care of the Elderly: Meeting the Challenge of Dependency, Academic Press, London
Fentonlewis A (1981) Fracturing the femur: changing incidence. British Medical Journal Z: 1217–1220
Fernie G R, Gryffe C I, Holiday P J, Llewellyn A 1982 The relationship of postural sway in standing to the incidence of falls in geriatric subjects. Age and Ageing 2: 11–17
Fine W 1959 An analysis of 277 falls in hospital. Gerontologia Clinica 1: 291–300
Fine W 1972 Geriatric ergonomics. Gerontologia Clinica 14: 322–332
Gray B 1966 Home accidents among old people. Royal Society for the Prevention of Accidents, London
Grimley-Evans J, Prudham D, Wandless, 1979 A prospective study of fractured femur: incidence and outcome. Public Health, London 93: 235–241
Gryfe C I, Amies A, Ashley M J 1977 A longi .dinal study of falls in an elderly population 1. Incidence and mortality. Age and Ageing 6: 201–210
Hakim A, Adams R D 1965 Journal of Neurological Sciences 2: 307–310
Hinsdale G 1887 Journal of Medical Sciences 93: 478
Isaacs B 1982 Balance and imbalance in old age. Advanced Medicine Conference. Pitman Medical 231–239
Leake W E 1964 Home accidents in a London suburb. The Medical Officer 112: 139–143
Lucht U 1971 A prospective study of accidental falls and resulting injuries in the home among elderly people. Acta Socio-medica Scandinavica 1: 105–120
Morfitt J M 1979 Accidents to old people in residential homes. Public Health, London 93: 177–184
Morris E, Isaacs B 1980 The prevention of falls in a geriatric hospital. Age and Ageing 9: 181–185
Naylor R, Rosen A J 1970 Falling as a cause of admission to a geriatric unit. The Practitioner 205: 327–330
Over R 1966 Possible visual factors in falls in old people. Gerontologist 6: 212–214
Overstall P W, Exton-Smith A N, Imms F J, Johnson A L 1977 Falls in the elderly related to postural imbalance. British Medical Journal 1: 261–264
Overstall P W 1978 Falls in the elderly — epidemiology, aetiology and management. In: Isaacs B (ed) Recent advances in geriatric medicine I. Churchill Livingstone, Edinburgh, ch 4, p61–72
Overstall P W, Johnson A L, Exton-Smith A N 1978 Instability and falls in the elderly. Age and Ageing Supplement 7: 92–95
Prudham D, Grimley-Evans J 1981 Factors associated with falls in the elderly: a community study. Age and Ageing 10: 141–146
Purdon-Martin J 1967 The basal ganglia and posture. Pitman, London
Rodstein M 1964 Accidents among the age. Journal of Chronic Diseases 17: 515
Sheldon J H 1948 The social medicine of old age. Report of an Inquiry in Wolverhampton. Nuffield Foundation, Oxford University Press
Sheldon J H 1960 On the natural history of falls in old age. British Medical Journal 2: 1685–1690
Sheldon J H 1963 The effect of age on the control of sway. Gerontologia Clinica 5: 129–138

Stevens D L, Matthews W B 1973 Cryptogenic drop attacks: an affliction of women. British Medical Journal 1: 439–442
Wild D, Isaacs B, Nayak U S L 1980 Report to DHSS. Department of Geriatric Medicine, University of Birmingham
Wild D, Nayak U S L, Isaacs B 1981a Facts on falling. Health and Social Services Journal 1413–1415
Wild D, Nayak U S L, Isaacs B 1981b How dangerous are falls in old people? British Medical Journal 282: 266–268
Wild D, Nayak U S L, Isaacs B 1981c Prognosis of falls in old people at home. Journal of Epidemiology and Community Health 35, 3: 200–204
Wild D, Nayak U S L, Isaacs B 1981d Description, classification and prevention of falls in old people at home. Rheumatology and Rehabilitation 20: 153–159
Witkin H A, Warpner S 1966 Possible visual factors in falls in old age. Gerontologist 212–214
Wollner L 1978 Managing postural hypotension: four effective lines of treatment. Modern Geriatrics 16–22
Wright B M 1971 A simple mechanical ataxia-meter. Proceedings of the Physiological Society 218: 27–30
Wyke B 1979 Cervical articular contributions to posture and gait: their relation to senile disequilibrium. Conference on the Ageing Brain Age and Ageing 8: 251–256

9
Peter Sandercock and Charles Warlow

The prevention of stroke in the elderly

INTRODUCTION

> There is little to suggest that the devastating consequences of stroke will be ameliorated by more expert medical or surgical management of the completed stroke. A more fruitful approach is to deal with its precursors rather than to delay until ... the stroke has already occurred.
> (Kannel & Wolf, 1983)

Most strokes result, directly or indirectly, from atheromatous disease of either the cerebral or coronary arteries. Atheroma may begin early in life, but there is usually a long incubation period before it becomes symptomatic. Symptoms from coronary disease tend to appear first in middle age; symptoms from cerebral arterial disease and strokes come later, becoming increasingly common in old age. Measures to prevent stroke may therefore need to start in the middle years of life or earlier and be continued into senescence if they are to succeed. Futhermore, since stroke is a common disease, a 'mass disease', individual doctors dealing with a few 'high-risk' patients can only make a relatively small contribution towards reducing the burden of stroke on the community (Rose, 1981). Long-term mass programmes are therefore needed, as well as the efforts of individual doctors, if stroke is to be prevented. Such programmes can only be undertaken if they are national, safe, simple and acceptable to the public. This chapter hopes to identify the elements of a preventive strategy which might fulfil these criteria.

DEFINITIONS

Clinicians generally have little difficulty in making a diagnosis of stroke when at the bedside, yet do not find it so easy to agree on a definition of stroke when sitting down to plan their research. Each new study appears to generate a new definition of stroke. With increasing knowledge, new subdivisions of the clinical and pathological varieties keep appearing, thus further complicating the issue. The commonest terms used to described the clinical varieties of stroke are, in order of increasing duration of symptoms: transient ischaemic attack (TIA), reversible ischaemic neurological deficit (RIND), minor stroke, partial non-progressing stroke, stroke in evolution, and completed stroke. TIA and stroke are the only two that are of relevance to this chapter.

Stroke

One of the simplest and most widely used definitions of stroke is the one devised by the WHO: Stroke is defined as rapidly developing clinical signs of focal, and at times global (applied to patients in deep coma and to those with subarachnoid haemorrhage), loss of cerebral function, with symptoms lasting more than 24 hours or leading to death, with no apparent cause other than vascular (Hatano, 1976).

Stroke can be further divided into three main pathological categories: cerebral infarction, primary intracerebral haemorrhage and subarachnoid haemorrhage. Epidemiological definitions of these terms are given in the paper on the incidence of stroke in Oxfordshire (Oxfordshire Community Stroke Project, 1983). In addition, there are at least five important subcategories of cerebral infarction: lacunar infarction, atherothrombotic infarction (ABI), infarction caused by emboli from the heart, haemorrhagic infarction and 'boundary zone' infarction. There is also a long list of unusual non-atheromatous diseases causing stroke (Barnett, 1980) but they are of limited relevance to the mass prevention of stroke because of their rarity.

TIA

The WHO definition is cumbersome, so Warlow & Morris (1982) have proposed the following: An acute loss of focal cerebral or ocular function, with symptoms lasting less than 24 hours, which after adequate investigation is presumed to be due to embolic or thrombotic vascular disease.

These definitions of stroke and TIA are simple and clear, but they obscure the complex, variegated nature of cerebrovascular disease. Caplan (1983) wryly sums up the difficulties: 'After all, these terms simply tell us how badly off the patient is; they say nothing about the mechanism of stroke. None of these categories approaches homogeneity; they contain fruits as divergent as grapes and watermelons.'

Are all these different types of strokes really important, since most of them are just different patterns of a single underlying process, namely atherosclerosis and hypertension? The answer is not clear at present, but in formulating a rational plan for the prevention of stroke, we should at least be aware that a single preventive measure may not prevent all types of stroke.

THE SIZE OF THE PROBLEM CREATED BY STROKE

Mortality from stroke

Mortality statistics derived from death certificates have three virtues; they are routinely collected in most countries, they are easily accessible and they cover large numbers of events over long periods of time. Unfortunately for cerebrovascular disease research, they also have several drawbacks, all of which reduce their accuracy. Death may occur years after the event, and the certifying doctor may forget to write 'stroke' on the certificate, even when it may have been a contributory cause of death. Even if 'stroke' does appear on the certificate, the clinical diagnosis of cerebral haemorrhage versus cerebral infarction is more likely to be wrong than right (Cameron & McGoogan, 1981).

Stroke is the third commonest cause of death in Britain; in 1982, 69 028 people were certified as dying from cerebrovascular disease (OPCS, 1983). Between 1950 and 1974, stroke mortality in England and Wales fell by 15–20 per cent, and by 32 per cent in the USA; Acheson & Williams (1980) have reviewed the possible reasons. The three most likely explanations are:
1. A fall in the incidence of stroke (i.e. fewer new cases per year)
2. A reduction in the case fatality rate of stroke (i.e. reduced risk of dying from the complications of stroke, such as pneumonia, say because of better antibiotics)
3. A systematic change in certification habits of doctors (e.g. transference of deaths to heart disease)

Death from stroke is therefore only a rough barometer of the problems created by the disease, and furthermore, as Muir Gray has suggested in the introduction, is perhaps not relevant anyway, since our aim is to prevent morbidity rather than death.

The incidence and prevalence of stroke

By contrast to mortality statistics, data on the incidence of stroke are not routinely collected, usually cover short periods of time and record relatively few events (and all epidemiologists abhor small numbers). The reasons for this are simply that incidence studies of stroke are hard work, expensive and cannot usually be done by clinicians in the course of their everyday clinical duties.

Practical problems and sources of bias in incidence studies

There are three main sources of bias in cerebrovascular disease incidence studies: failure to find all the cases (incomplete ascertainment), incorrect clinical diagnosis and failure to determine the pathological type of stroke in every case. Complete ascertainment of all new cases, both at home and in hospital, is vital to ensure the sample is representative and not biased towards the more serious cases managed in hospital. This may be particularly difficult when measuring the incidence of TIA, since some patients undoubtedly do not contact their doctors, even though they may be having repeated attacks.

Correct clinical diagnosis of stroke is not always easy, and studies which rely on questionnaire responses or retrospective searches of medical records are likely to be very inaccurate (Brewis et al, 1966). Wiebers & Whisnant (1982) suggested that all cerebrovascular surveys should ideally be based on a diagnosis made by a neurologist at the time of the event.

Finally, it is vital that the pathological type of stroke be determined in every case by X-ray computerised tomography of the head (CT scan) or postmortem. It is important to realise that even the prestigious Framingham study, until the advent of CT scanning, could not reliably distinguish cerebral infarction from haemorrhage, since their definition of cerebral infarction stipulated only that the CSF should be free of blood (Dawber, 1980). The CT scan shows primary intracerebral haemorrhage sufficiently often in patients with bloodless CSF (Ruff & Dougherty, 1981) and in those with a cardiac source of embolism (Sandercock et al, 1984), that any study which has not verified the pathological type by CT scan or postmortem may be seriously biased. Such bias could easily obscure the relationship between a given risk factor and a particular type of stroke.

Short-term studies on the incidence of stroke

Our own study of stroke in a representative sample of patients, which used a neurologist for clinical diagnosis and obtained a CT scan or postmortem in 89 per cent of cases, has recently been published (Oxfordshire Community Stroke Project, 1983). In the first year of the study 168 cases of stroke were registered; 76 per cent were due to cerebral infarction (of which about a quarter were 'lacunar'), 13 per cent intracranial haemorrhage, and in 11 per cent the pathological type was not known. Table 10.1 gives the age-and sex-specific incidence rates, which rise steeply with age; half the cases are aged over 75. The frequency of stroke in a given population will therefore depend mainly on its age structure, so if incidence rates are to be compared in different populations, they must be 'age-adjusted' to a standard population. If these figures are so adjusted, the annual rate in the 1981 England and Wales population would be 1.96 per 1000 population per year. This would give an estimated 96 000 new cases of stroke each year in England and Wales. Kurtzke (1983) quoted similar figures for incidence rates around the world. He also calculated the prevalence of stroke (number of survivors of stroke alive on 'prevalence' day divided by the number of people in the population on that day) to be about 6 per 1000 population in most Western countries; Weddell & Beresford (1979), over a four-year observation period, calculated that the prevalence of stroke in Frimley, UK, was similar. It is important to stress the three most important factors which can increase prevalence: increased disease incidence rate, increased average survival after onset and lengthening the period of observation.

Longitudinal studies of stroke incidence

The Mayo Clinic is the only centre which has been able to monitor the

Table 9.1 Yearly age-and sex-specific incidence rates per 1000 for first stroke (Oxfordshire Community Stroke Project, 1983) (reproduced with permission from the British Medical Journal)

Age	No. of cases/No. at risk	Males Rate	95% confidence interval
0–54	7/ 41 999	0.17	0.04– 0.29
55–64	15/ 4 710	3.18	1.58– 4.79
65–74	20/ 3 360	5.95	3.35– 8.55
75+	32/ 1 797	17.82	11.69–23.9

Age	No. of cases/No. at risk	Females Rate	95% confidence interval
0–54	6/ 38 797	0.16	0.03– 0.28
55–64	14/ 4 796	2.92	1.39– 4.45
65–74	26/ 3 776	6.89	4.25– 9.52
75+	48/ 3 379	14.21	10.22–18.20

Age	No. of cases/No. at risk	Males + Females Rate	95% confidence interval
0–54	13/ 80 796	0.16	0.07– 0.25
55–64	29/ 9 506	3.05	1.94– 4.16
65–74	46/ 7 136	6.45	4.59– 8.30
75+	80/ 5 175	15.46	12.10–18.82
Total	168/102 613	1.64	1.39– 1.88

incidence of stroke with a reasonable degree of accuracy in a defined population (Rochester, Minnesota) over a prolonged period. Garraway et al (1979) reported a decline in Rochester, not only in stroke incidence, but also in both cerebral haemorrhage and cerebral infarction, over the period 1945 to 1974. Anderson & Whisnant (1982) compared mortality rates in the Rochester population with those in the USA as a whole for the same period. They found that Rochester death certificate diagnoses were very accurate. Mortality rates from stroke were always lower in Rochester than in the USA as a whole, and the rate declined in both, by 12 per cent in the USA, and by 67 per cent in Rochester, over the 20-year study period. The authors concluded that the decline of mortality in both populations was not an artefact and was probably mainly due to the falling incidence of stroke. There are many possible factors which might be responsible for the decline in incidence, such as improved treatment of hypertension, successful early modification of other risk factors and a trend to a healthier lifestyle in the general US population. Unfortunately, the epidemiological data on whether it is these or other, as yet unidentified, factors which are responsible, falls tantalisingly short of proof.

Long-term surveillance of stroke incidence in a few well-organised centres around the world, despite its enormous cost, is clearly an important part of any mass prevention programme. The World Health Organisation is now coordinating a series of such studies (1982).

The incidence and prevalence of TIA

TIAs are generally infrequent and, by definition, do not result in impairment or disability. Though they are quite common and are an important risk factor for stroke (see 'TIA as a risk factor'), they are often not recognised or treated before the stroke occurs. Patients may sometimes ignore transient episodes of limb paraesthesiae or weakness, or perhaps attribute them to 'arthritis' or 'neuritis'. Such misconceptions may also lead to the general practitioner making an incorrect diagnosis. There are other diagnostic pitfalls — episodes of transient monocular loss of vision (amaurosis fugax) may be diagnosed as 'migraine', or subtler manifestations of cerebral ischaemia as 'hypertension', which may delay effective treatment.

The incidence of TIA in the community is therefore difficult to measure. The best large study of TIA incidence is based on the community of Rochester, Minnesota. Whisnant et al (1976) found the average annual incidence of first attacks of TIA was 0.31 per 1000, with age-specific rates rising with age to 3 per 1000 over the age of 75. Choosing a prevalence day at the end of a fifteen-year observation period, they calculated a point prevalence rate of 1.5 per 1000 population (patients with a first attack of TIA at some time in the preceding 15 years, surviving free of stroke to prevalence day divided by the number of people in the population alive on that day). The age-specific point prevalence in those aged 65 and over was 1.8 per 1000.

THE EFFECTS OF STROKE

Physical problems after stroke

This subject has been investigated by several large studies (Marquardsen, 1969; Harris, 1971; Weddell & Beresford, 1979; and Brocklehurst, Andrews & Morris, 1980) and has been recently reviewed by Anderson (1982) and Langton-Hewer (1983).

Definition and measurement

Like the definition of stroke, the number of different definitions of physical difficulties after stroke and their measurement nearly equals the number of publications on the subject. Fortunately, most workers in the field now seem to agree that Harris's (1971) definitions of impairment, disability and handicap should be regarded as definitive.

Cerebrovascular disease creates some unique problems for those trying to measure the associated physical problems. The patients are elderly, and many already have a variety of impairments as a result of normal ageing, such as poor vision, loss of memory, reduced hearing and impaired cognitive function. Other common physical problems such as osteoarthritis, ischaemic heart disease and frequent falls, may make it difficult to decide whether the stroke has added anything to the existing background level of impairment.

Furthermore, in the acute phase the deficit may fluctuate rapidly, from hour to hour, and from day to day, as changing blood pressure, hydration, cerebral blood flow and intercurrent infection alter cerebral function. As recovery proceeds, fatigue, depression, loss of motivation and recurrent stroke may cause continuing variations in performance.

The Barthel scale (Barthel & Mahoney, 1965) seems to have overcome at least some of these problems and has proved to be a simple, repeatable and valid measurement of physical disability in stroke patients. A score is derived from the patient's actual performance in activities of daily living (ADL), rather than from an assessment of what the patient is felt able to do; the difference between these two is important (Barthel & Mahoney, 1965, Labi et al, 1980).

Physical problems and recovery from stroke

Marquardsen (1969) identified and meticulously followed a large hospital-based series of 769 stroke patients. He found that of those who survive the first weeks after stroke, 52 per cent were restored to independence in self-care, 15 per cent became able to walk again, but needed some help with personal needs, and 33 per cent never regained independence for either self-care or walking. Weddel & Beresford (1979), in a community-based sample of stroke patients, surprisingly found quite similar results. Of those surviving to four years (only 20 per cent of the original sample) 78 per cent were independent for transfers, 80 per cent were able to walk out of doors, and 90 per cent were being cared for in their own homes. Langton-Hewer (1983) reviews these problems, and the prevention of disability after stroke, in more detail.

The quality of life after stroke and its measurement

If measuring physical difficulties after stroke is difficult, trying to assess the damage done to the stroke sufferer's quality of life is even more hazardous. After a stroke, depression, irritability, feelings of hopelessness, isolation and loss of self-esteem are all common. There are well-validated methods for assessing some of these psychological problems, such as the General Health Questionnaire for general psychiatric morbidity (Goldberg & Hiller, 1979), and the Hamilton (Hamilton, 1960) and the Zung (Zung, 1965) rating scales for depression. These scales are well suited to younger people without physical impairments, but may prove quite inappropriate in many elderly stroke patients. Better methods of measuring these important problems in elderly stroke patients are needed.

Labi et al (1981) studied 121 long-term survivors of stroke who had all recovered to the point of being independent in all activities of daily living. All therefore achieved the best score possible on the Barthel and other ADL indices, yet one-third had not returned to their normal pre-stroke social activities. The authors were unable to determine the cause of this failure. It might have resulted from subtle disability that could not be detected by the Barthel score (i.e. the Barthel was too insensitive) or from social and psychological factors (such as fear of going out alone).

Robinson (1982) found in a selected series of 113 stroke patients that 30 per cent were depressed; depression seemed commonest between six and twelve months after stroke. Strokes affecting the left hemisphere appeared to be more frequently associated with depression than right-hemisphere strokes. These and associated problems are reviewed in detail by Brocklehurst (1980) and Anderson (1982).

SCOPE FOR PRIMARY PREVENTION

Risk factors for stroke and their treatability

Age

Age is the most powerful single risk factor for stroke (Kurtzke, 1983); the incidence rate of stroke rises logarithmically with age. All other risk factors are influenced by age, and most become less significant with increasing age. As mentioned in the introductory chapter, the 'rectangularisation of the age-at-death curve' suggests that medical progress has done little to influence the biological process of ageing: we are just better at enabling people to survive into senescence. However, we should not be defeatist about the apparently inexorable nature of ageing; though we may never learn how to *reverse* any of the factors that link ageing to stroke, we may at least learn how to *prevent* some of them.

Blood pressure in the middle aged and risk of stroke

Studies in many countries have shown that high arterial blood pressure is a risk factor for stroke in both sexes, in many different races and irrespective of whether other risk factors are present or not (Kurtzke, 1983). The higher the level of either systolic or diastolic pressure measured in middle age, the higher is the risk of all forms of stroke in subsequent years (Dawber, 1980). The gradient of risk is steeper for systolic than for diastolic pressure. There is no clear 'threshold' level below which risk is no longer related to pressure, and thus there is no absolute distinction between 'normal' and 'abnormal' blood pressure (Grimley Evans & Rose, 1977). Nonetheless, the Framingham study found that if 160/95 mmHg was taken as the dividing line between 'hypertension' and 'normotension', then a middle-aged person with 'hypertension' was three times more likely to have a stroke due to atherothrombotic brain infarction (ABI) in the next 24 years than someone with 'normotension' (Dawber, 1980).

Comparing the risk of ABI between those with the highest (> 180 mm Hg) and the lowest (< 120 mm Hg) systolic pressures, the ratio of risk was 8:1 (this is known as the *relative* risk). Fortunately, there are few people in the general population who are at such high risk of stroke. This high risk group therefore contributes only a small number of strokes to the total number of new cases of stroke in the community. There are, however, as many as a million people in Britain with a phase V diastolic pressure of > 105 mm Hg, and perhaps a further three million people with phase V diastolic pressures between 100 and 104 mm Hg (Anon, 1980 a) at more modest risk of stroke. Many strokes will occur in this 'modest-risk' group, simply as a result of its very large size.

Thus the majority of the cases of stroke in the community which result from the effects of hypertension (the population *attributable* risk) come not from the few at high risk, but from the many exposed to low risk. This principle is central to any strategy for the prevention of stroke (Rose, 1981), and is further illustrated in the example derived by him from the Veterans Administration study of mild–moderate hypertension in men (1972) (Table 9.2).

Two-thirds of the attributable coronary deaths and three-quarters of the attributable deaths from stroke occur in men with phase V diastolic pressures below 110 mm Hg, and about half the attributable coronary deaths and a quarter of the attributable deaths from stroke occur below 100 mm Hg. This example highlights the importance of a community-based approach to the detection and treatment of mild to moderate hypertension in the prevention of stroke.

Treating hypertension in middle-aged people. The treatment of hypertension should begin at a level above which the effects of investigation and treatment do more good than harm. The level may be affected by factors such as age and sex and by personal and cultural assessments of 'good' and 'harm' (Grimley Evans & Rose, 1977). There have been thirteen randomised controlled studies of sufficient size to address this question: there have been five studies in asymptomatic people (i.e. no evidence of hypertension related disease) — Hamilton et al (1964), Smith (1977), Johnson et al (1978), Management Committee (Australian Study, 1980), Helgeland (1980); five in mixed populations of symptomatic and asymptomatic patients — Wolf & Lindeman (1966), Veterans Administration (1970, 1972), Barraclough et al

Table 9.2 Population attributable mortality from coronary heart disease and stroke arising at different levels of blood pressure (reproduced with permission from the British Medical Journal and Professor Rose)

Diastolic BP	Cumulative percentage of excess deaths attributable to hypertension	
	Coronary heart disease	Stroke
< 80	0	0
< 90	21	14
< 100	47	25
< 110	67	73
> 110	100	100

(1973), Hypertension and Detection Follow up Program (HDFP) (1979, 1982 a, 1982 b); two in survivors of stroke — Carter (1970), and Hypertension-Stroke Cooperative Study Group (1974); one in the elderly — Sprackling et al (1981). Three important studies on the treatment of hypertension in the elderly are still in progress — The European Working Party on Hypertension in the Elderly (Amery & de Schaeparijver, EWPHE, 1973), the Medical Research Council Study on Mild Hypertension (MRC, 1977) and Coope (1983).

All of the published studies have been reviewed in detail elsewhere — by Warlow (1982), Toth & Horwitz (1983) and Mitchell (1983) among others.

These studies have shown that drug treatment of moderate to severe hypertension (phase V diastolic BP >105 mm Hg, +/− systolic BP > 160 mm Hg), in both males and females under the age of 65, significantly reduces the risk of stroke and death, though it does not appear to reduce the incidence of myocardial infarction so much. The trails only contained small numbers of patients over 65, and therefore no firm statements can be made about benefits in this age group. Treatment appears to be more effective if hypertension-related 'end-organ damage' such as ischaemic stroke or e.c.g. evidence of left ventricular hypertrophy (LVH) is present. Drug treatment appears least effective in those with 'mild' hypertension (phase V diastolic below 105 mm Hg) and no evidence of end-organ damage, and those aged under 50 with 'mild' hypertension (Veterans Administration, 1972; Management Committee (Australian study), 1980).

The costs and benefits of drug treatment of mild hypertension

The available trials suggest that drugs can lower the risk of stroke in some people with phase V diastolic blood pressures between 90 and 104 mm Hg. If this result is extrapolated to the population of Britain, we must consider treating perhaps three million people with antihypertensive agents (Anon, 1980 a). The likely benefits of such a policy have been calculated by Mitchell (1983) using the results from the Australian trial (Table 9.3).

The benefit is clear — treatment prevented 14 strokes (31−17). The costs are that 104 171 people were screened to find the subjects for the study

Table 9.3 How much benefit from treating hypertension at how much cost? (reproduced with permission from Butterworths and Professor J.R.A. Mitchell)

	Active group ($n=1721$)	Placebo group ($n=1706$)
Strokes despite therapy	17	
Strokes on placebo		31
Potential strokes prevented	14	
Patients treated to achieve this	1704	
Patients remaining stroke-free despite no therapy		1675

(though screening 52 000 people would have found enough for the 'active' group), and 1704 people took drugs unnecessarily as it turned out. The risks to those on drug therapy, though small, create a large population-attributable risk because of the large numbers treated, and have been reviewd (Rose, 1981; Gill & Beevers, 1983); symptoms such as loss of wellbeing (I felt all right until I started taking the tablets), lassitude, postural dizziness, and impotence in males are common. Biochemical abnormalities (raised urea, urate, impaired glucose tolerance, and hypokalaemia on diuretics, raised lipids on beta-blockers) though asymptomatic, may ultimately *increase* the risk of stroke or heart attack (Veterans Administration, 1972; MRC, 1977; MRFIT, 1982; Arnesen et al, 1983).

Huth & Torwitz (1983) conclude from their review that the results of the published trials of mild hypertension are of more relevance to those concerned in deciding on public health policy than to family doctors deciding on how to treat individual patients.

Are non-drug treatments the answer to mass hypertension? Blood pressure may fall by a few mm Hg in people who lose weight, take more exercise, take up meditation or relaxation exercises, stop smoking and reduce their intake of salt and saturated fat (Anon, 1980 b; Beared et al, 1982; Puska et al, 1983). If this small reduction occurred in a very large number of people, the reduction in the population risk of stroke attributable to hypertension might be large (Rose, 1981; Gill & Beevers, 1983). Rose (1981) calculated that the life-saving benefits of all current antihypertensive therapy might be equalled by a downward shift of the blood pressure distribution curve of the entire population by 2–3 mm Hg. To back up this suggestion, there is evidence that the enthusiasm of the American population for a healthier lifestyle has contributed to their decline in cardiovascular mortality (MRFIT, 1982); Britons have not as yet followed suit quite so energetically. It will be a great challenge to find the cheapest, yet most effective and ethical ways of encouraging Britons in the same direction.

Hypertension and risk of stroke in the elderly

The relationship between level of blood pressure and stroke becomes more complex in old age. Systolic and diastolic pressures rise with age until about the seventh decade, when they may fall again (Grimley Evans & Rose, 1977). Blood pressure becomes more variable in old age. One to three readings of blood pressure in a middle-aged person may be enough to get a very accurate assessment of 'blood-pressure related risks' (Dawber, 1980). In an elderly person, many more readings may be necessary before these risks can be accurately measured (Grimley Evans et al, 1980). Cardiovascular diseases which may lower blood pressure, yet are in themselves associated with increased risk of stroke and death, such as myocardial infarction and atrial fibrillation, are common in the elderly, and may further distort the 'risk/blood pressure' relationship.

Furthermore, since the damaging effects of hypertension on the vascular system may be cumulative with time, *duration of hypertension* might be a much more relevant measurement in the elderly than *current level* of blood pressure. 'End points' that one might use in studies on the effects of blood pressure in the elderly are also more difficult to assess. For example, a non-fatal stroke causing slight weakness and clumsiness of one arm and leg might easily pass unnoticed in someone with severe arthritis, but cause the patient to fall and fracture her femur. Failure to detect such a stroke might then mean that these two causes of significant morbidity would not be attributed to the effects (direct or indirect) of hypertension; in other words, hypertension would appear less dangerous than it really is. Since such non-fatal events may be difficult to detect in the elderly, many studies use death as the end point instead, yet, as I emphasised earlier, this is not always a particularly relevant end point: we are trying to prevent *morbidity* rather than *mortality*.

These difficulties are reflected in the literature. Fry (1970) reported that hypertension was not a risk factor for stroke in a small number of elderly patients in his general practice. In 1974, Shekelle, Ostfeld & Klawans reported that in a group of patients aged 65–74 blood pressure greater than 160/95 mm Hg did carry a slightly increased risk of stroke (relative risk of 1.8). Kannel et al (1980) found in the Framingham study that systolic hypertension remained an important risk factor for stroke up to age 75; their data were inadequate to be certain about the risk in older patients. Grimley Evans et al (1980), in a well-designed study in the over 65s, found no relationship between blood pressure and either morbidity or mortality. Miall & Brennan (1981) found that, although there was a significant relationship between systolic pressure and cardiovascular mortality for those aged over 65, this did not hold for those aged 75 and over (Peart, 1981). Rajala et al (1983) found an *inverse* relationship between blood pressure and mortality in a small group aged over 85. Coope (1983) pointed out that this might be due to some confounding variable which might lower blood pressure and increase mortality, and cited data from his own study, to confirm this possibility. Patients with conditions such as atrial fibrillation, heart failure and diabetes mellitus are excluded from his controlled study of hypertension in the elderly. Cardiovascular deaths among the hypertensives are 10.8 per cent compared with 5.2 per cent in the non-hypertensives; thus if patients with conditions likely to lower blood pressure are excluded, the relationship between blood pressure and cardiovascular disease is restored, even in the elderly. A further study by Garland et al (1983) tends to confirm this.

In conclusion, evidence is accumulating that hypertension is not benign in the elderly, and carries an increased risk of stroke and death. This does not mean that hypertension *should* be treated in the elderly; only the results of randomised controlled trials can tell us whether the benefits of doing so outweigh the risks (O'Malley & O'Brien, 1980).

Threshold for drug treatment in the elderly. This has not been clearly established for patients aged over 65. The trials in progress should give considerable guidance. In the meantime, only one reasonably satisfactory study has been published (Sprackling et al, 1981), which showed that in a group of patients, 83 per cent of whom were aged over 74, drug treatment of hypertension (phase IV diastolic > 100 mm Hg) did not reduce mortality (morbidity was not measured) over the next four years.

TIA as a risk factor for stroke

TIA are said to occur before 10–72 per cent of ischaemic strokes; case selection and retrospective recall of transient events are likely to increase the percentage in many of the reported series; the true figure is probably between 10 and 25 per cent. Schoenberg et al (1980) found that TIA carry a relative risk of stroke of 4.6; only hypertension carried a higher risk (relative risk 6). The risk of stroke after TIA is approximately 7 per cent per annum, or in other words, after five years about one third of all TIA patients will have had a stroke.

Medical treatment of TIA and the prevention of stroke. There is some debate on whether treatment of patients with TIA should be considered primary or secondary prevention; the difference is arbitrary and I shall not mention it further. The medical management of patients after TIA has been thoroughly reviewed by Genton et al (1977), Barnett (1980) and Warlow (1982). In essence, TIA carries the same risk factors for stroke, so management of hypertension, hyperlipidaemia and other risk factors is important in patients with TIA. Debate now revolves around two main questions:
1. Should 'antiplatelet' agents be used, and if so which (and in what dose)?
2. Is carotid endarterectomy of any value in patients with TIA, stroke and even those with aysmptomatic carotid stenosis?

Aspirin and stroke prophylaxis. There has been only one large randomised controlled trial of aspirin and sulphinpyrazone therapy after TIA (Canadian Cooperative Study Group, 1978). This study showed that sulphinpyrazone was no better than placebo, and that aspirin in a dose of 325 mg q.d.s appeared to reduce the risk of stroke. This effect was more obvious in men than women, but such a subgroup analysis might, by chance, have come up with the wrong answer. Other subsequent trials have been smaller and prone to type 2 statistical errors (demonstrating no statistically significant difference between two different treatments, when a small but important difference dose exist). The pooled results from all of the other randomised trials would be compatible with those of the Canadian trial, namely that aspirin might reduce the risk of stroke and/or death after TIA by 25–30 per cent (Peto R, personal communication). None of these studies have yet answered three important questions:
1. Does aspirin benefit women *at all?*
2. Does aspirin increase the risk of cerebral haemorrhage?
3. What would be the risk to the community if aspirin were used on a national scale in the primary prevention of stroke?

For some of the answers we must await the results of three important trials:

1. The UK-TIA aspirin study of placebo versus 300mg aspirin daily versus 1200 mg aspirin daily, which has so far randomised 2200 patients (more than all published studies combined). It should be completed by 1987.

2. The British doctors' study, which was randomly allocated 5000 healthy male British doctors to '500 mg aspirin daily' or 'avoid aspirin if possible'. The study will be reporting its findings in 1985.

3. The American doctors' study, which has randomly allocated 21 000 American physicians to one of four regimes: aspirin 325mg per 48 hrs, carotene, aspirin + carotene, or no therapy. This study will report its findings in the early 1990s.

These studies should clarify the risk–benefit ratio of aspirin therapy in primary prevention of stroke, TIA and myocardial infarction, though they will provide only limited data on secondary prevention of stroke. Studies on the latter are much needed.

A rough risk–benefit ratio for widespread aspirin therapy can be calculated using data from the Canadian trial. Only half of all the new cases of first attack of TIA in the community are likely to be eligible for aspirin therapy, because of dyspepsia, peptic ulceration, aspirin sensitivity, old age, or because they are already on a preparation likely to interact adversely with aspirin (e.g. warfarin, non-steroidal anti-inflammatory agents etc.). If we assume that treatment reduces the annual risk of stroke and/or death by 25 per cent from 10 to 7.5 per cent per year over five years, the expected results would be as shown in Table 9.4. The incidence of non-fatal myocardial infarction would probably also be reduced (Anon, 1980c). There might be further unexpected benefits, such as reduced formation of cataracts which has recently been reported (Bennett, 1983).

If we assume the incidence of side-effects to be the same as in the Canadian study (in which a quarter of the patients were also taking sulphinpyrazone), then perhaps 800 patients might have suffered 'heartburn', and between 30 and 250 might have had significant gastrointestinal bleeding (Bennett, 1983).

Carotid endarterectomy to prevent stroke? Stenotic and ulcerated atheromatous lesions at the origin of the internal carotid artery in symptomatic and

Table 9.4 How much benefit from aspirin therapy at how much cost?

New cases of first TIA per year*	21 651
Eligible for aspirin therapy	10 285
Number of strokes/deaths after five years**	4 211
Number of strokes/deaths after five years' aspirin therapy***	3 320
Approximate number of strokes prevented over five years	891
Patient-years of 'unnecessary' aspirin-taking	40 946

*In England and Wales 1981 population, unpublished data from OCSP
**Stroke and/or death at 10%/year
***Stroke and/or death at 7.5%/year

asymptomatic patients carry an increased risk of stroke. Surgery to remove such lesions would seem an attractive way to reduce that risk and, indeed, carotid endarterectomy is being performed more frequently, particularly in North America (Warlow, 1984). However, though the operation itself carries a significant risk of stroke, none of the vascular surgeons who claim to have a low operative mortality have definitely demonstrated that the risk of surgery is less than that of no surgery. In a review of the subject, Warlow (1984) concludes that there is certainly no evidence in favour of, or against, the operation. He makes a plea that the operation only be done as part of satisfactory randomised controlled trials so that current trials can be completed as quickly as possible. Only then can we formulate a national policy for the proper use of this expensive, risky and yet potentially useful operation.

The British, French and Dutch Collaborative Study of Carotid Endarterectomy, which began in 1981, is a randomised trial designed to address this question, but does not expect to be able to show a significant difference between the treatment groups until 1987 at the earliest.

If the current trials do conclude that carotid endarterectomy in patients with TIA and mild ischaemic stroke improves their prognosis, how many people might be eligible? Only a small and highly variable proportion of all TIA patients in Britian undergo carotid angiography, and an even smaller proportion undergo carotid endarterectomy (UK-TIA Aspirin Study Group, 1983). Warlow (1984) estimates that perhaps 5000 patients (all ages) might be eligible for surgery in England and Wales per year, yet fewer than 1000 actually have the operation. Successful surgery for these patients could produce a very worthwhile reduction in stroke incidence, though the cost would be high; a detailed cost–benefit analysis would be very useful.

Heart disease as a risk factor for stroke

Coronary artery disease (CAD). Coronary artery disease is a risk factor for stroke (Friedman, 1968; Schoenberg, 1980; Dawber, 1980; Kurtzke, 1983), and for ABI (Dawber, 1980; Kurtzke 1983). In the Framingham study, the presence of CAD increased the risk of ABI threefold; if congestive cardiac failure was also present, the relative risk was increased to 9.

Atrial fibrillation. Friedman et al (1968) found atrial fibrillation (AF) six times more often among a series of elderly stroke patients than in a group of controls matched for age, sex and blood pressure. In the Framingham study, Wolf et al (1978) found that AF, in the absence of rheumatic heart disease (RHD), increased the risk of stroke fivefold, and in the presence of RHD, increased the risk 17-fold. It is presumed that a thrombus forms in the fibrillating left atrium and that fragments break off it, resulting in cerebral embolism and stroke. However, it is almost impossible in life, and can be difficult even at postmortem, to prove that a given patient in AF has a stroke as a result of embolism from the left atrium. Despite considerable technical advances in the methods of non-invasive cardiac imaging in patients with ischaemic stroke (Donaldson, Emanuel & Earl, 1981), they are still unreliable at detecting left atrial thrombus. In Wolf's study, left atrial thrombus as found in only one case at postmortem.

The relationship between AF and stroke becomes more tenuous when other variables are taken into account. AF is associated with other risk factors for stroke, notably hypertension (Kannel, et al, 1982), and perhaps it is often just a marker for hypertensive heart disease, rather than a direct cause of the stroke. Furthermore, AF is common, particularly in the elderly, and its prevalence increases with age, occurring in 5 per cent of those aged over 75 (Campbell, Cird & Jackson, 1974). However, it would seem logical that at least patients in AF and proven left atrial thrombus should be treated with anticoagulants. Before we vigorously pursue such a policy, it would be wise to know the answers to the following questions:
1. Is non-rheumatic AF really a risk factor for stroke?
2. If so, is it also a risk factor for stroke in the elderly?
3. Can a reliable method be found to detect left atrial thrombus?
4. Are anticoagulants safe in the elderly patient in AF?

Other forms of heart disease and stroke. Lesions such as mitral regurgitation, mitral valve prolapse (MVP), mitral annulus calcification (MAC) and hypertrophic obstructive cardiomyopathy are all said to be associated with an increased risk of stroke. Rarer conditions such as subacute bacterial endocarditis and embolism from prosthetic heart valves also carry an increased risk of stroke. The relevance of these and other lesions to stroke has been reviewed by Genton et al (1977), Barnett (1980) and de Bono (1984), among others. It is difficult to be certain of the population risk of stroke attributable to these lesions; further results from the Oxfordshire Community Stroke Project may be useful in this respect. It is unlikely that the risk will be large.

Anticoagulants for patients in AF and with other heart lesions? Given the uncertainty about the relevance of these various cardiac lesions to ischaemic stroke, the diversity of opinion on the value of anticoagulant therapy is hardly surprising. The relevant trials have all been discussed in the reviews mentioned in the previous section. At present, anticoagulants should be reserved for younger patients with rheumatic heart disease, mitral stenosis with AF, artificial valve prostheses, recent myocardial infarction and one or two other rarer cardiac conditions. Large randomised trials are needed before a rational treatment policy can be formulated for the elderly patient with non-rheumatic atrial fibrillation (Sage & van Uitert, 1983; de Bono, 1983; Starkey & Warlow, 1984). 'Anti-platelet' drugs such as aspirin may have some part to play in the management of some of these cardiac lesions but, again, further trials are needed (see Warlow, 1982).

Smoking

Smoking appears to carry only a small excess risk of stroke. Salonen et al

(1982) found that in Finnish men aged under 50, smoking carried a fourfold excess risk of stroke. In the Framingham study, Kannel (1983) reported that the risk was marginal and confined to men aged under 65. The excess risk of stroke due to smoking was independent of other risk factors in both studies. Deubner (1980) calculated that eliminating the effects of smoking from the population of Evans County, Georgia, would produce a 10 per cent reduction in cardiovascular mortality (though most of the deaths prevented would be from heart disease rather than from stroke). Giving up smoking *after* a stroke is unlikely to reduce the risk of subsequent stroke for the average patient, and may just increase the misery.

Increased haematocrit

Both polycythaemia rubra vera and raised haematocrit within the range of normal carry an increased risk of stroke (Kannel, 1983). In the latter group, the effect is reduced when the effects of smoking and hypertension are allowed for. Raised haematocrit is also associated with reduced cerebral blood flow (Thomas et al, 1977). The level of the haematocrit may correlate with the size of cerebral infarcts (Harrison et al, 1981). Pearson & Wetherly-Mein (1978) showed that venesection to reduce haematocrit in primary polycythaemia appeared to reduce the risk of vascular occlusive episodes. Wade (1983) showed that venesection in patients with secondary polycythaemia increased both cerebral blood flow and cerebral oxygen delivery. It is not known whether venesection in secondary polycythaemia reduces the risk of stroke.

Obesity

Kurtzke (1983) felt that obesity was not a major risk factor for stroke. Nonetheless, weight reduction in the middle aged may be an important part in a primary preventive strategy. The aim should be a general shift of the mean weight-for-height curve of the whole population, rather than spectacular weight loss for a few very obese individuals as recommended in the Report of a Subcommittee of The Royal College of General Practitioners (RCGP) Working Party on Prevention (RCGP, 1981).

Diabetes mellitus

Diabetes mellitus is an important independent risk factor for ABI: even allowing for such associated factors as raised cholesterol, the relative risk of ABI is 2 (Kannel, 1983). Though evidence is beginning to accumulate that tight control of glycaemia may reduce the incidence of some of the vascular complications of diabetes, there is no evidence as yet that ABI is reduced. Furthermore, the relatively low prevalence of diabetes in the community means that the population risk of stroke attributable to diabetes is small.

Deubner (1980) calculated that the removal of the effects of diabetes from the population of Evans County, Georgia, would reduce the ten-year cardiovascular mortality rate by only 4 per cent.

Lipids

'The relationship of serum cholesterol to atherothrombotic brain infarction in the Framingham data was always somewhat equivocal. After 24 years' observation this is still the case' (Dawber, 1980). A week effect was seen in men under the age of 50. Deubner (1980) calculated that removing the effects of hypercholesterolaemia from the Evans County population might reduce ten-year cardiovascular mortality by 4 per cent. The WHO trial of clofibrate demonstrated that achieving even such a small, but potentially worthwhile, benefit has its costs. Clofibrate did reduce cholesterol and cardiovascular mortality, but at the cost of increased non-vascular deaths (Committee of Principal Investigators, 1980). Salonen et al (1982) have reported that raised triglycerides increase the risk of both brain infarction and other strokes by a factor of about 2.5 in men; there was no increase in women.

Socioeconomic status and stroke

In 1978, Acheson reviewed the relation of socioeconomic status to cerebrovascular mortality rates in different parts of Britian. He found a marked inverse relationship; low status and manual occupation were invariably associated with a standardised mortality ratio greater than 100 for cerebrovascular disease. The gradient was steepest for cerebral thrombosis. Salonen, Puska & Tuomilehto (1982) found that in men, not only low socioeconomic status but unmarried status and urban residence also carried an increased risk of death from stroke. Further data from incidence studies are needed to clarify the relationship.

Diet and water hardness

Dietary intake of many factors such as salt, calcium (in relation to water hardness), managesium, potassium, trace elements and vitamins have all been related to the incidence of stroke. Space must limit discussion to two topics of recent interest.

Acheson (1978, 1980 and 1983) has suggested that the inverse relationship between social class and stroke might, in part at least, be due to low intake of vitamin C in social class V. He cited biological evidence that vitamin C deficiency might predispose to stroke. A prospective study in Norway by Vollset & Bjelke (1983) has also shown that low vitamin C intake may be a risk factor for stroke. Acheson's proposal (1983) that encouraging an increased intake of fresh fruit and vegetables in the general population would not be harmful and might reduce to incidence of stroke, seems reasonable, and should now be tested more directly.

Water hardness appears to have an inverse relationship to cardiovascular mortality. Chin et al (1978) reviewed the evidence for such a relationship for stroke in Britain, and found the data inadequate. The British Regional Heart Survey (Pocock et al, 1980) has yet to publish its final report, but in their preliminary communication the authors suggested that regional variations in cardiovascular mortality could be explained by variations in five factors. These were: water hardness, rainfall, temperature, and two social factors (percentage of manual workers and car ownership). The effect of water hardness on cardiovascular mortality was independent of the other four factors.

Physical activity

Paffenbarger & Wing reported (1967) that, in a cohort of 50 000 male Harvard alumni, those who had participated in varsity sports while at college had a mortality rate from fatal stroke half that of non-participants. The Framingham study (Dawber, 1980) showed a benefit of more modest levels of exercise to men who were aged 50–59 at entry to the study. In Finland (Salonen, Puska & Tuomilehto, 1982), low physical activity at work in men and women was associated with an increased risk of stroke, myocardial infarction (MI) and death from all causes. Low physical activity during leisure time only increased the risk of death, but not MI or stroke. More work needs to be done in this field before a really clear picture emerges as to who will benefit most from how much physical activity.

Season and climate

Chin (1980) and Kurtzke (1983) have reviewed the associations between temperature, admission to hospial with stroke, and death from stroke. They both concluded that there does seem to be a U-shaped relationship, with maxima at both extremes of temperature. Further studies in this area will be interesting, in view of the recently demonstrated variations in population blood pressure with temperature (Brennan et al, 1983). If temperature-related swings in blood pressure are a common precipitant of stroke, then one simple but expensive preventive measure might be to install central heating in every elderly person's house.

Alcohol

Alcohol intake, especially binge drinking, may be a risk factor for stroke in the young (Anon, 1983). Evidence from the British regional heart study suggests that alcohol intake, particularly heavy drinking, may be an important risk factor for stroke and MI in Britain. If this is proven, then it will add increasing weight to the pressure for a government-sponsored campaign to reduce alcohol consumption in Britain (RCGP, 1981; Deitch, 1983).

MULTIPLE RISK FACTORS AND IDENTIFYING THOSE AT HIGHEST RISK

The risk factors for stroke interact in such a way that a single risk factor, such as blood pressure, should never be considered in isolation (Madhavan & Alderman, 1981). For example, a person with a systolic blood pressure of 135 mm Hg may be at greater risk of stroke than someone of the same age with a pressure of 195 mm Hg, as a result of their smoking or serum cholesterol levels (Madhavan & Alderman, 1981). Nonetheless, an estimate of an individual's future risk of cardiovascular disease (not stroke) may be calculated roughly from measurements of just five variables, which are: serum cholesterol, blood pressure, e.c.g., smoking history and a test of glucose tolerance (Kannel, McGee & Gordon, 1976). The resulting risk score's usefulness is based on the dangerous assumption that the patient's constitution is similar to the average person in the Framingham cohort. It does not take account of factors such as TIA, which might be very important in a 'stroke risk' score. Nonetheless, it is the best currently available. Patients at highest risk of cardiovascular disease may be identified and treated accordingly, thus avoiding unnecessary treatment of those at low risk.

This approach was used in a large trial (Multiple Risk Factor Intervention Trial Research Group, 1982), in which 13 866 men aged 35 to 57 were recruited. Entry criteria were that the subjects should be at increased risk of coronary artery disease (CAD), but have no clinical evidence of it. They were categorised as high risk if their levels of three risk factors, namely serum cholesterol, smoking habit and blood pressure, were such that they were in the top 15 per cent of a risk score derived from the Framingham data. They were then randomised to receive a special intervention (SI) programme designed to reduce the levels of all risk factors, or to their usual sources of medical care (UC). Over the following seven years, against a background of falling mortality from CAD in the USA as a whole, the incidence of CAD was less than expected in both the SI and UC group. The trend was for less CAD and stroke mortality in the SI group, though it never reached statistical significance. There are many possible explanations for this marginal result. One is that the UC group actively reduced their levels of risk factors much more than expected, and therefore reduced any differences between UC and SI. Another explanation is that various measures in the SI group, such as some of the antihypertensive agents used, may have *increased* mortality in selected subgroups in SI.

The lessons from this study for doctors in the NHS are difficult to see clearly, since the MRFIT results are much more applicable to the American health care system than our own. The study does at least suggest that risk factor intervention might reduce the risk of stroke. A modified system of identifying high-risk patients could be developed to suit the needs of British general practitioners. Furthermore, general practitioners would then be in an ideal position to provide the long-term treatment follow-up which is so important for success. Plans for the prevention of atherosclerotic disease by general practitioners have been formulated (RCGP, 1981), but these may need to be refined to deal specifically with the problem of stroke.

THE COSTS OF STROKE

In Britain, about 50 per cent of patients are admitted to hospital shortly after their stroke. Once in hospital, they may stay there for very long periods. In Scotland in 1976, patients with cerebrovascular disease used 1 070 998 bed days, which was 11 per cent of all hospital bed days in all specialties (excluding mental illness and maternity) (Carstairs, 1976). Patients managed at home use few resources (Weddell & Beresford 1979; Garraway et al, 1980). The most frequently used, and the most useful, was the home help service. Garraway also observed that the allocation of resources related neither to functional performance of the patients, nor to their probable need for those services. He made a plea that clearer criteria for providing services be established.

It is difficult to sum up all the costs of stroke, both direct and indirect. Carstairs (1976), allowing for direct health costs only, estimated that stroke consumed 5 per cent of all health resources in Scotland. Hartunian, Smart & Thompson (1980) allowing for indirect costs such as loss of earnings, as well as direct health costs, calculated that stroke was the fourth costliest disease in the USA (after cancer, heart disease and motor accidents), costing $6.5 billion in 1975. Of course these figures reveal nothing of how *usefully* this money was spent; Garraway's results suggest that a lot of it could probably have been spent much more effectively.

CONCLUSIONS

1. Stroke can be prevented by the 'mass' approach.
2. The 'mass' approach to stroke prevention will require some, if not all, of the following:
a. A downward shift of the nation's blood pressure distribution.
b. Perhaps a downward shift of the nation's weight distribution.
c. Perhaps various alterations in the nation's diet, such as reduced fat content and increased vitamin C intake.
d. Campaigns to reduce alcohol and tobacco consumption.
3. General practitioners should continue identifying and treating 'high-risk' patients.
4. More research is needed, in particular into:
   a. Improving methods to identify those at highest risk of stroke which are

applicable in general practice.
b. Randomised trials of the value of the following treatments:
   i. hypertension in the elderly
   ii. anticoagulants for patients in atrial fibrillation
   iii. venesection for those with raised haematocrit
   iv. aspirin in secondary prevention of stroke
   v. carotid endarterectomy

REFERENCE

Acheson R M, Sanderson C 1978 Strokes: social class and geography. Population Trends 12: 13–17
Acheson R M, Williams D R R 1980 Epidemiology of cerebrovascular disease: some unanswered questions. In: Rose F C (ed) Clinical neuroepidemiology. Pitman Medical, Tunbridge Wells
Acheson R M, Williams D R R 1983 Does consumption of fresh fruit and vegetables protect against stroke? Lancet 1: 1191–1193
Amery A, de Schaeparijver A 1973 European working part on high blood pressure in the elderly (EWHPE): organization of a double-blind multicentre trial on antihypertensive therapy in elderly patients. Clinical Science and Molecular Medicine 45: 715–735
Anderson G L, Whisnant J P 1982 A comparison of the trends in mortality from stroke in the United States and Rochester, Minnesota. Stroke 13: 804–809
Anderson R 1982 The aftermath of stroke. Department of Health and Social Security, London
Anon 1980 a Millions of mild hypertensives. British Medical Journal 281: 1024–1025
Anon 1980 b Lowering blood pressure without drugs. Lancet 2: 459–461
Anon 1980 c Aspirin after myocardial infarction. Lancet 1: 1172–1173
Anon 1983 Binge drinking and stroke. Lancet 2: 660–661
Arnesen E, Thelle D S, Forde O H, Mjos O D 1983 Serum lipids and glucose concentrations in subjects using antihypertensive drugs: Finnmark 1977. Journal of Epidemiology and Community Health 37: 141–144
Barraclough M et al 1973 Control of moderately raised blood pressure: report of a cooperative randomised controlled trial. British Medical Journal 3: 434–436
Barnett H J M 1980 Progress towards stroke prevention: Robert Wartenburg lecture. Neurology 30: 1212–1224
Barthel D W, Mahoney F I 1965 Functional evaluation: the Barthel index. Maryland State Medical Journal 14: 61–65
Beard T C, Gray W R, Cooke H M, Barge R, 1982 Randomised controlled trial of a no-added sodium diet for mild hyptertension. Lancet 2: 455–458
Bennett A 1983 The future for aspirin. MIMS Magazine November 15: 28–29
Brennan P J, Greenberg G, Miall W E, Thompson S G, 1982 Seasonal variation in blood pressure. British Medical 285: 919–923
Brewis M, Poskanzer D C, Rolland C, Miller J 1966 Neurologiical disease in an English city. Acta Neurologica Scandinavica (Supplementum 24) 24: 47
Brocklehurst J C, Andrews K, Morris P E 1978 Medical, Social and psychological aspects of stroke in elderly patients. Final report. University of Manchester Department of Geriatric Medicine, Manchester
Cameron H M, McGoogan E 1981 A prospective study of 1152 hospital autopsies: I. Inaccuracies in death certification. Journal of Pathology 133: 273–283
Campbell A, Caird F I, Jackson T F M, 1974 Prevalence of abnormalities of electrocardiogram in old people. British Heart Journal 36: 1005–1011
Canadian Co-operative Study Group 1978 A randomized trial of aspirin and sulphinpyrazone in threatened stroke. New England Journal Of Medicine 299: 53–59
Caplan L R 1983 Are terms such as completed stroke or RIND of continued usefulness? Stroke 14: 431–433
Carstairs V 1976 Stroke: resource consumption and the cost to the community. In: Gillingham F J, Mawdsley C, Williams A E, (eds) Stroke. Proceedings of the ninth Pfizer international symposium. Churchill Livingstone, London

Carter A B, 1970 Hypotensive therapy in stroke survivors. Lancet 1: 485–489
Chin P L, Angunawela R, Mitchell D, Horne J 1980 Stroke register in Carlisle: a preliminary report. In: Rose F C (ed) Clinical neuroepidemiology. Pitman Medical, Tunbridge Wells
Committee of Principal Investigations 1980 Report of a WHO cooperative trial on primary prevention of ischaemic heart disease using clofibrate to lower serum cholesterol — mortality follow-up. Lancet 2: 379–384
Coope J R 1983 High blood pressure and mortality in the elderly. Lancet 2: 746
Dawber T R 1980 The Framingham study: the epidemiology of atherosclerotic disease. Harvard University Press, Cambridge, Mass
de Bono D P 1984 Do anticoagulants prevent embolism from the heart to the brain? In: Warlow C P, Garfield J (eds) Dilemmas in the management of the neurological patient. Churchill Livingstone, Edinburgh
Deitch R 1983 Alcoholism: a Government-sponsored right? Lancet 2: 409–410
Deubner D C, Wilkinson W E, Helms M J, Tyroler M A, Hames C G, 1980 Logistic model estimation of death attributable to risk factors in Evans County, Georgia. American Journal of Epidemiology 112: 135–143
Donaldson R M, Emanuel R W, Earl C J 1981 The role of two-dimensional echocardiography in the detection of potentially embolic intracardiac masses in patients with ischaemic stroke. Journal of Neurology, Neurosurgery and Psychiatry 44: 803–809
Friedman G D, Loveland D B, Ehrlich S P 1968 Relationship of stroke to other cardiovascular disease. Circulation 38: 533–541
Fry J 1974 Natural history of hypertension: a case for selective non-treatment. Lancet 2: 431
Garland C, Barrett-Connor E, Suarez L, Criqui M H 1983 Isolated systolic hypertension and mortality after age 60 years: a prospective population-based study. American Journal of Epidemiology 118: 365–376
Garraway W M, Walton M S, Akhtar A J, Prescott R J 1981 The use of health and social services in the management of stroke in the community: results from a controlled trial. Age and Ageing 10: 95–104
Garraway W M, Whisnant J P, Furlan A J, Phillips L H, Kurland L T, O'Fallon W M 1979 The declining incidence of stroke. New England Journal of Medicine 300: 499–452
Genton E, Barnett H J M, Fields W S, Gent M, Hoak J C 1977 XIV. Cerebral ischemia: the role of thrombosis and antithrombotic therapy. Stroke 8: 150–175
Gill J S, Beevers D G 1983 Hypertension and wellbeing. British Medical Journal 287: 1490–1491
Goldberg D F, Hiller V F 1979 A scaled version of the General Health Questionnaire. Psychological Medicine 9: 139–145
Grimley Evans J, Rose G 1977 Hypertension. British Medical Bulletin 27(1): 37–41
Grimley Evans J, Prudham D, Wandless I 1980 Risk factors for stroke in the elderly. In: Barbagallo-Sangiorgi G, Exton-Smith A N (eds) The ageing brain — neurological and mental disturbances. Plenum, New York
Hamilton M 1960 A rating scale for depression. Journal of Neurology, Neurosurgery and Psychiatry 23: 56–62
Hamilton M E N, Thompson E N, Wisniewski T K M, 1964 the role of blood pressure control in preventing complications of hypertension. Lancet 1: 235–238
Harris A I 1971 Handicapped and impaired in Great Britain. Office of Population Censuses and Surveys. Social Survey Division, London
Harrison M J G, Kendall B E, Pollock S, Marshall J 1981 Effect of haematocrit on carotid stenosis and cerebral infarction. Lancet 2: 114–115
Hartunian N S, Smart C N, Thomson M S, 1980 The incidence and economic cost of cancer, motor vehicle injuries, coronary heart disease and stroke: a comparative analysis. American Journal of Public Health 70: 1249–1260
Hatano S, Experience from a multicentre stroke register: a preliminary report. Bulletin of the World Health Organization 54: 541–553
Helgeland A, Treatment of mild hypertension: a five-year controlled drug trial — the Oslo study. American Journal of Medicine 69: 725–732
Holbrook M, Skilbeck C E, 1983 An activities index for use with stroke patients. Age and Ageing 12, 166–170
Hypertension Detection and Follow-up Program Group 1979 Five-year findings of the Hypertension Detection and Follow-up Program: I Reduction in mortality of persons with high blood pressure, including mild hypertension. Journal of the American Medical Association 242: 2562–2571

Hypertension Detection and Follow-up Program Cooperative Group 1982 a The effects of treatment on mortality in mild hypertension: results of the Hypertension Detection and Follow-up Program. New England Journal of Medicine 307: 976–980 Hypertension Detection

Hypertension Detection and Follow-up Program Cooperative Group 1982 b Five year findings of the Hypertension Detection and Follow-up Program: III Reduction in stroke incidence among persons with high blood pressure. Journal of the American Medical Association 247: 633–638

Hypertension–stroke Cooperative Study Group 1974 Effect of antihypertensive treatment on stroke recurrence. Journal of the American Medical Association 229: 409–418

Johnson H B, Pearce V R, Hamilton M 1978 Treatment of mild hypertension — an attempted controlled therapeutic trial. Journal of Chronic Diseases 31: 513–519

Kannell W B, Wolf P A 1983 Epidemiology of cerebrovascular disease. In: Ross Russell R W (ed) Vascular disease of the central nervous system 2nd edn, Churchill Livingstone, London

Kannell W B, McGee D, Gordon T 1976 A general cardiovascular risk profile: the Framingham study. American Journal of Cardiology 38: 46–51

Kannell W B, Abbott R D, Savage D D , McNamara P M 1982 Epidemiologic features of atrial fibrillation: the Framingham study. New England Journal of Medicine 306: 1018–1022

Kannell W B L Wolf P A, McGee D L, Dawber T R, McNamara P, Castelli W P 1980 Systolic blood pressure, arterial rigidity and risk of stroke. The Framingham study, Journal of the American Medical Association 245: 1225–1229

Kurtzke J F 1983 Epidemiology and risk factors in thrombotic brain infarction. In: Harrison M J G, Dyken M L (eds) Cerebral vascular disease Butterworth, London

Labi L C, Phillips M S, Gresham G E 1980 Psychosocial disability in physically restored long-term survivors of stroke. Archives of Physical Medicine and Rehabilitation 61: 561–565

Langton-Hewer R 1983 Stroke rehabilitation. In: Ross Russell R W (ed) Vascular disease of the central nervous system 2nd edn. Churchill Livingstone, Edinburgh

Madhavan S, Alderman M H 1981 The potential effect of blood pressure reduction on cardiovascular disease. A cautionary note. Archives of Internal Medicine 141: 1583–1586

Management Committee 1980 The Australian therapeutic trial in mild hypertension. Lancet 1: 1261–1267

Marquardsen J 1969 The natural history of acute cerebrovascularr disease: a retrospective survey of 769 patients. Munksgaard, Copenhagen

Medical Research Council Working Party on Mild to Moderate Hypertension 1977 Randomised controlled for mild hypertension: design and pilot trial. British Medical Journal 1: 1437–1440

Miall W E, Brennan P J 1981 In: Onesti G, Kim K E (eds) Hypertension in the young and old. Grune & Stratton, New York

Mitchell J R A 1983 Hypertension and stroke. In: Harrison M J G, Dyken M L (eds) Cerebral vascular disease. Butterworth, London

Multiple Risk Factor Intervention Trial Rearch Group 1982 Multiple risk factor intervention trial: risk factor changes and mortality results. Journal of the American Medical Association 248: 1465–1477

Office of Population Censuses and Surveys 1983 OPCS Monitor. October: 1–3

O'Malley K, O'Brien E 1980 Management of hypertension in the elderly. New England Journal of Medicine 302: 1397–1401

Oxfordshire Community Stroke Project 1983 Incidence of stroke in Oxfordshire: first year's experience of a community stroke register. British Medical Journal 287: 713–717

Paffenbarger R S, Wing A L 1967 Characteristics in youth predisposing to stroke in later years. Lancet 1: 753–754

Pearson T C, Wetherly-Mein G 1978 Vascular occlusive episodes and venous haematocrit in primary proliferative polycythaemia. Lancet 2: 1219–1222

Peart W S, Miall W E, Greenberg G, Meade T 1981 Blood pressure reduction in the elderly. British Medical Journal 283: 1397

Pocock S J, Shaper A G, Cook D G, Packham R F, Lacey R F, Powell P F, Russell P F 1980 British regional heart survey: geographic variations in cardiovascular mortality and the role of water quality. British Medical Journal 280: 1243–1249

Puska P, Nissinen A, Vartainen E, Dougherty R, Mutanen M, Iacomo J M, et al 1983 Controlled randomised trial of the effect of dietary fat on blood pressure. Lancet 1: 1–9

Rajala S, Haavisto M, Heikinheimo R, Mathla R 1983 Blood pressure and mortality in the very old. Lancet 1: 520–521

Robinson R G, Price T R, 1982 Post-stroke depressive disorders: a follow-up of 103 stroke patients. Stroke 13: 635–641

Rose G 1981 Strategy for prevention: lessons from cardiovascular disease. British Medical Journal 282: 1847–1851
Ross Russell R W (ed) Vascular disease of the central nervous system, 2nd edn. Churchill Livingstone, Edinburgh
Royal College of General Practitioners 1981 Prevention of arterial disease in general practice RCGP, London
Ruff R L, Dougherty J H, 1980 Evaluation of acute cerebral ischemia for anticoagulant therapy: computed tomography or lumbar puncture. Neurology 31: 736–740
Sage J I, van Uitert R L 1983 Risk of recurrent stroke in patients with atrial fibrillation and non-valvular heart disease. Stroke 14: 537–540
Salonen J T, Puska P, Tuomilehto J 1982 Physical activity and risk of myocardial infarction, cerebral stroke and death: a longitudinal study in eastern Finland. American Journal of Epidemiology 115: 516–537
Salonen J T, Puska P, Tuomilehto J, Homan K 1982 Relationship of blood pressure, serum lipids and smoking to the risk of cerebral stroke: a longitudinal study in eastern Finland. Stroke 13: 327–333
Sandercock P A G, Warlow C P, Starkey I R, Molyneux A J 1984 The value of routine C T scanning and echocardiography in the assessment of acute stroke. Journal of Neurology, Neurosurgery and Psychiatry 47, 420
Schoenberg B S, Schoenberg D G, Pritchard D A, Lilienfield A M, Whisnant J P 1980 Differential risk factors for completed stroke and transient ischemic attacks (TIA). Transactions of the American Neurological Association 105: 165–167
Shaper A G, Pocock S J, Walker M, Cohen M, Wale C J, Thompson A G 1981 British regional heart survey: cardiovascular risk factors in middle-aged men in 24 towns. British Medical Journal 283: 179–186
Shekelle R B, Ostfield A M, Klawans H L 1974 Hypertension and the risk of stroke in an elderly population. Stroke 5: 71–75
Smith W M 1977 U S Public services Co-operative Study Group. Treatment of mild hypertension: results of a ten year intervention trial. Circulation Research 40 (suppl 1): 180–187
Sprackling M E, Mitchell J R A, Watt G 1981 Blood pressure reduction in the elderly — a randomised controlled trial of methyldopa. British Medical Journal 283: 1151–1153
Starkey I R, Warlow C P 1984 Long-term anticoagulation for the fibrillating stroke patient? Archives of Neurology (In press)
Thomas D J, Marshall J, Ross Rusell R W, Wetherly-Mein G, Du Boulay G, Pearson T C et al Effect of haematocrit on cerebral blood flow in man. Lancet 2: 941–943
Toth P J, Horwitz R I 1983 Conflicting trials and the uncertainty of treating mild hypertension. American Journal of Medicine 75: 482–483
UK-TIA Study group 1983 Variation in the use of angiography and carotid endarterectomy by neurologists in the UK-TIA aspirin trial. British Medical Journal 286: 514–518
Veterans Administration Co-operative Study Group on Antihypertensive Agents 1970 Effects of treatment on morbidity in hypertension: II results in patients with diastolic blood pressure averaging 90 through 114 mm Hg. Journal of the American Medical Association 213: 1143–1152
Veterans Administration Co-operative Study Group on Antihypertensive Agents 1972 Effects of treatment on morbidity in hypertension. Circulation 45: 184–194
Vollset S E, Bjelke E 1983 Does consumption of fruit and vegetables protect against stroke? Lancet 2: 742
Wade J P H 1983 Transport of oxygen to the brain in patients with elevated haematocrit values before and after venesection. Brain 106: 513–523
Warlow C 1984 Carotid endarterectomy — does it work? Stroke (in press)
Warlow C, Morris P J (eds) 1982 Transient ischemic attacks. Dekker, New York
Wedell J, Beresford S A A 1979 Planning for stroke patients: a four year descriptive study of home and hospital care. HMSO, London
Whisnant J P 1976 A population study of stroke and TIA: Rochester, Minnesota. In: Gillingham F J, Mawdsley C, Williams A E (eds) Stroke: proceedings of the ninth Pfizer international symposium. Churchill Livingstone, Edinburgh
Wiebers D O, Whisnant J P 1982 Epidemiology. In: Warlow C, Morris P J (eds) Transient ischemic attacks. Dekker, New York

Wolf F W, Lindeman R D 1966 Effects of treatment in hypertension: results of a controlled study. Journal of Chronic Diseases 19: 227–240
Wolf P A, Dawber T R, Kannell W B 1978 Heart disease as a precursor of stroke. In: Schoenberg B S (ed) Advances in Nuerology, vol 19. Raven Press, New York
World Health Organization 1982 MONICA Newsletter 1: 1–8
Zung Z W K 1965 A self-rating depression scale. Archives of General Psychiatry 12: 63–70

10   *Elaine Murphy*

Prevention of depression and suicide

DEPRESSION — THE EXTENT OF THE PROBLEM

Depression in old age is commonly regarded as a predictable, understandable, though sad response to the losses and declines of the last period of life. The themes of old age and depression have often been linked as if inevitably entwined. Samuel Johnson, for example, expressed this in 'Vanity of Human Wishes' (1749):

> That life protracted is protracted woe.
> Time hovers o'er, impatient to destroy
> And shuts up all passages of joy.

This is essentially a younger man's pessimistic view of the gloomy outlook for old age. We know now that the majority of elderly people do not feel depressed, unhappy or unfulfilled and that the fear and hopelessness which many young people feel about their future years is mainly a result of stereotyped misconceptions. For every older person who feels life in old age is worse than they expected in their youth, there are three others who believe life has turned out better than they expected (Morris, 1975). Nevertheless, significant and severe depression is common in old age. Sufferers endure a particularly distressing misery which not only blights their own lives but has far-reaching consequences for the morale of those around them. In its severest form, depression is one of the most disabling mental illnesses, and a substantial proportion of the workload of psychiatric services for the elderly consists of providing treatment and care for the depressed.

Depression is unfortunately a word in common currency. The lay person's view of being 'depressed' is simply being 'sad', 'fed up' or 'bored'. Psychiatrists, on the other hand, talk confidently of 'depressive illness', a syndrome in which persistently lowered mood is accompanied by physiological symptoms such as weight loss, insomnia, psychomotor retardation and subjective loss of concentration. For the psychiatrist, depressive illness becomes 'depressive psychosis' when guilt feelings, delusional ideas and severe hypochondriasis complicate the picture. At the milder end of the spectrum, depression is indistinguishable from the sadness and demoralisation which most individuals go through at some stage of their lives in response to unhappy circumstances; at the other end, depressive psychosis may be a life-threatening and disabling illness.

The truth is that, in most doctors' experience, the majority of depressed elderly people fall on a continuum somewhere between these two extremes and do not fit conveniently into 'illness' or 'no illness'. This has led to enormous problems in comparing the results of epidemiological studies, since what has been included in one study as a 'case' may be very different from a 'case' in another study. The results of prevalence studies, both in the USA and UK, of depression in elderly people living in the community have varied widely from 2 per cent (Bollerup, 1975) up to 60 per cent (Leighton, 1963).

The major difficulty has been to find a reliable method of case identification which can be replicated by other workers. However, three recently published studies have partially solved the problem by using interview schedules administered by highly-trained interviewers in which each symptom was scored using detailed and explicit criteria. The results of these studies allow a comparison of symptom counts between different populations. Alternatively, it is possible to impose arbitrary cut-off points to designate a 'case' or 'non-case'. Using similar, but not identical methods, Blazer and Williams, in North Carolina (1980), Gurland, New York (1980) and Weissman and Myers, New Haven (1978) produced point prevalence rates of between 8 per cent and 14 per cent for depression in community residents of 65 years and over. In all three studies, depression 'cases' were judged to be at a clinical level of severity which warranted attention from medical services. All three studies found a prevalence rate of 1–2 per cent for depressive psychosis of a severity likely to require treatment in hospital.

However, the picture may be different in the very old, that is those over 75 years. Community surveys have hitherto excluded elderly people living in institutions. Although the overall proportion of elderly people in old people's homes is small, about 4 per cent in the USA and UK, this figure rises to 8 per cent for the over-75-year-olds. The residents of these institutions are the group at highest risk of physical and psychiatric illness. The prevalence rate of psychiatric disorder in old people's homes in the UK has been variably estimated at between 30 and 50 per cent. Hence, the exclusion of this group from population surveys is likely to lead to an underestimation of the overall prevalence of depression in the eldlery.

Point prevalence studies taken from a cross-section of the population tend to assume that differences in prevalence rates at different ages are due to the effects of the ageing process itself. However, cohorts of elderly people from different generations may have markedly different prevalence rates. We are witnessing now the ageing of those born before World War 1 who grew up in a culture very different from our own. The mental health of future generations of elderly people may show a different pattern. There is already evidence that the rise in suicide rates of young people in many Western societies, which first began about 30 years ago and has continued with successive birth cohorts, may remain with the cohort as the group ages (Solomon & Hellon, 1980; Murphy & Wetzel, 1980). Klerman (1976) speculated that today's youth, ageing in the twenty-first century, may perhaps complain more of neurotic depression and seek treatment for it, maintaining the attitudes and demands of their current culture for early treatment of uncongenial mood states. Future generations of elderly may therefore require a different style of psychiatric practice. The changing pattern of depression over the last fifty years is only too clear from Lewis's classic descriptions of 'melancholia' written in 1936. The deluded, retarded *young* patients whom he described are rarely seen in psychiatric practice nowadays, but the case descriptions are immediately recognisable to psychiatrists working with the elderly as being typical of certain of today's elderly depressed patients.

A further point about depression rates is worthy of consideration. At all ages, women are more likely to suffer from depression than men. However, after the age of 70 years, the rate among men begins to rise (Gurland, 1976), although it never quite catches up with that for women. Finally, it should be noted that in the oldest subjects of all, the 85- and 90-year-olds, there is some suggestion that those who survive in the community have a lower rate of depression compared with 60- and 70-year-olds. This is likely to be an artefact produced by the removal into institutions of a high proportion of the frail among the oldest generation, but it is possibly also a reflection of the indomitable personal characteristics of the oldest survivors of all who are still managing in their own homes.

THE EFFECTS OF THE PROBLEM

For the purposes of this chapter, the term 'depression' is used to denote a clinical syndrome which not only affects mood but interferes with the ability to think and concentrate, and impairs sleep and appetite. Depression of this kind is commoner than dementia. Only in the over-85-year-old age group does the prevalence of dementia rise above that of depression. Forty per cent of all new referrals to a comprehensive psychiatric service for the elderly in East London are for treatment of depression (Murphy, 1982).

In spite of this large referral rate, the majority of depressed patients are not admitted to hospital. However, the small proportion who are admitted to hospital for treatment use a large part of the services for the elderly (Jolley & Arie, 1976). This is not only because of the high overall total incidence of new cases in a large elderly population, but because of the high relapse rate after first discharge. Two-thirds of all admissions for depression in this age group are readmissions. In a recent study of the use of beds by depressed elderly patients over a four-year period, a quarter of the total number of acute psychiatric beds available for all age groups was used by the elderly (Murphy & Grundy, 1984).

The serious nature of depression is emphasised by the high mortality rate.

Kay (1962) reported that the mortality rate over a two-and-a-half-year period following first admission to hospital for treatment was double that expected. Kay's patients all had affective disorder presenting for the first time in old age. In particular this author noted a higher than expected rate of deaths from cerebrovascular disease.

More recently, Murphy (1983) reported a 19 per cent mortality rate for men and 11 per cent for women in the first year of follow-up of 124 depressed elderly patients. Murphy included both inpatients and those treated as day patients and at home, and also included patients who had a history of previous depressive episodes in younger life. The expected mortality rate over the course of a year was 5 per cent for both sexes, when the age and sex distribution of the group was taken into account. Thus the mortality rate for elderly depressed men was strikingly high and, although numbers were too small to analyse in depth, vascular disease seemed to be an important contributing cause, supporting Kay's notion that vascular disease and depression may be closely related in old age. It is possible that cerebrovascular pathology has a direct causal role in depression in old age or perhaps increases vulnerability to other causal agents. Alternatively, the physiological arousal which accompanies depression may lead to a rapid worsening of an already compromised cerebrovascular system. Both putative mechanisms warrant further study.

The mortality risk is also heightened by the risk of suicide. It is extremely difficult to estimate the overall risk of suicide in depression because, as will be noted later, few depressed elderly people are known by their family doctor to be depressed and even fewer receive treatment. Furthermore, suicides are often inaccurately registered, partly because of the very fact that there is no evidence of pre-existing depression reported at inquest. However, a review of the literature has suggested that, in depressed patients attending for psychiatric treatment, there is an overall lifetime risk of 15 per cent in those with recurrent depression, but with no history of mania (Guze & Robins, 1970). The risk is higher in older, physically ill men, and the issues involved are discussed later in this chapter.

Suicide risk among depressed patients is highest in the two years after first presenting for treatment. Murphy's one-year follow-up revealed only one suicide in 124 patients. However, there were also two deaths by self-starvation, inanition and subsequent pneumonia where there was no direct suicidal act but where the patients' determination to interfere with effective medical treatment to keep them alive might be construed as suicidal. Subsequent necropsy of these two patients revealed no other obvious serious illness.

Mortality rates and hospital admission rates for patients treated by psychiatrists reflect the problems posed by those with severe depressive illnesses. However, the vast majority of depressed elderly subjects are never referred to a psychiatrist and indeed are unlikely even to be known to their GP. Williamson (1964) reported that 71 per cent of elderly depressed subjects in the community were unknown to their family doctor. This proportion may have decreased over the past twenty years with the overall improvement in primary care services. However, little comfort is given on this score by Gruer's later study of a large sample of elderly people in the Scottish border counties. He found that, of the 42 per cent with psychological symptoms, half were not recorded in the GP's medical records as suffering from psychological symptoms, even though a high proportion of the sample had attended their GP withing the previous three months complaining of physical symptoms (Gruer, 1975). Older subjects with psychological symptoms are less likely to go to the doctor with their symptoms than younger people, though they might very well go with symptoms of physical illness masking a depression, and this is particularly true of older men (Goldberg. 1976).

Curiously at odds with these findings is the large number of prescriptions of psychotropic drugs given to the elderly. A study of one year's prescriptions by GPs in Oxfordshire reported that a third of elderly women and 20 per cent of elderly men received at least one prescription for a psychotropic drug at some point during the year (Skegg et al, 1977). It seems then that psychological symptoms are very likely to be treated by GPs with psychotropic drugs without any formal recognition of the diagnosis of depression.

Depression is such a commonly used term that it is as well to be reminded of the suffering and hardship endured by those afflicted. Patients often describe their feelings as 'a sense of being trapped', 'the future seems hopeless', 'a blank darkness ahead'. Emotions seem empty and shallow. The depressed subject finds it impossible to take an interest in children and grandchildren who were previously the focus of their lives. There is often an all-pervading feeling of desolation and irremediable emptiness. It is hard for relatives and friends to understand the self-preoccupation, withdrawal from social gatherings, the lethargy of hours wasted in purposeless inactivity while household chores are neglected. The sufferer often feels quite unable to participate in normal social interaction and, while clinging to the reassuring company of relatives, may yet drive them away by irritating and self-centred behaviour. Family and friends often feel neglected and rejected and begin to visit less frequently, finally leaving the patient feeling more socially isolated than ever. A depressed person is a depressing companion, and families need maximum help and support if they are to carrry on caring for the patient.

PREVENTABILITY

The primary prevention of mental illness preoccupied many workers in the early part of the twentieth century. Unfortunately there is little concrete evidence that successful preventive measures have been found. The child guidance movement started in the United States at the turn of the century with the expressed belief that many mental disorders of adulthood had their origins in faulty personality development arising from the mismanagement of children. Sadly, this early enthusiasm has not paid off in terms of preventing adult mental illness. Preventability depends on a thorough understanding of the aetiology, and we are not yet in that position with depression at any age. However, there are three groups of factors which appear to be of importance, and a thorough understanding of the mechanisms of interaction of these factors may ultimately lead to a coherent policy for primary prevention. The three groups of causal factors are, firstly, biological cerebral factors, secondly, physical health factors and, lastly, psychosocial factors.

Biological factors

Major affective psychoses at all ages occur in those who are genetically predisposed. However, the evidence for a strong genetic component is greatest in young people with bipolar manic depressive illness. In general, the older the patient at first onset of depression, the less likelihood there is of a positive family history. This may be due in part to the difficulty of obtaining a reliable history about parents' and grandparents' mental illnesses from an older subject. Mendlewicz (1976), reviewing evidence from a variety of studies, concluded that the genetic component was small for depression in old age.

There are, however, biological changes in the ageing brain which might make elderly people more vulnerable to depression. It has been known for many years that severe depression is associated with a depletion of biogenic amines in the brain. It has also been shown that catecholamines are lowered in the hindbrains of ageing animals and, postmortem, in patients who have died as a result of a range of illnesses. It has been tempting to assume that healthy subjects also have an age-related reduction of catecholamines in the brain. This reduction is hypothesised to cause a functional depletion of biogenic amines and thus predispose to depression. The case is, however, unproven. The biochemical basis of mood control is extremely complex, and so far we have no evidence that amine metabolism in the elderly is more susceptible to developing the biological changes which correlate with depression.

An alternative suggestion by Grauer (1977) was concerned with neurohumoral changes in old age. Diminishing thyroid function and decreased responsiveness of the pituitary to hypothalamic-releasing factors may make it more difficult for the aged to cope with stress. This interesting hypothesis warrants further study.

More importantly, there is evidence of neuro-physiological changes in elderly patients with depression. Hendrickson (1979) found a delay in the auditory evoked response on e.e.g. which was significantly greater in depressed elderly patients than for normal elderly controls but less than the delay in demented patients. The delay did not return to normal after recovery from the episodes of depression. This suggests that there may be biological cerebral changes that remain abnormal following recovery from depression. Jacoby & Levy (1980) studied a series of depressed elderly inpatients clinically and with computer tomogram scanning. There emerged a small sub-group with enlarged ventricles who differed clinically from other elderly depressed patients in being older, less anxious and having more physiological symptoms of depression, such as early-morning waking, weight loss, psychomotor retardation and so on. A follow-up study showed that this group had a high mortality rate. It must be stressed that these severely depressed patients do not show evidence of dementia or acute confusion. A further study demonstrated that brain tissue density, measured quantitively on the CT scan, was lower in depressed elderly compared with normal controls (Jacoby, 1983).

It is possible that the more severe forms of depression in old age are linked with cerebral pathology related to the ageing process but which is of a different nature from that occurring in dementia. Unfortunately, in our current state of knowledge, prevention of these biological changes is impossible. We must therefore look to other aetiological factors to institute preventive measures.

Physical illness

At all ages, physical ill health and depression are closely linked, but the relationship is especially marked in old age. This association has been demonstrated by many authors, notably Roth & Kay, (1956), Kay & Bergmann (1966) and Post (1969). The nature of the relationship was examined further by Murphy (1982) in a study comparing a wide range of possible aetiological factors in depressed patients with a comparison group of elderly people in the general population judged to be psychiatrically normal. The range of physical illness was rated along two separate scales. Firstly, the prevalence of chronic physical illness was noted on a six-point scale, the top three points reflecting chronic physical illness which either produced marked handicap in social functioning or seriously interfered with life expectancy. Secondly, sudden deteriorations of health were noted, these latter episodes being rated as 'adverse health life-events', for example, sudden onset of stroke, myocardial infarction or discovery of breast carcinoma requiring mastectomy.

The health of depressed patients was rated for a period of a year before first onset of depression and rated for the year before interview for the normal elderly. Twenty-six per cent of normal elderly had chronically poor physical health, compared with 39 per cent of depressed patients receiving psychiatric treatment. However, of depressed elderly subjects discovered during the course of the general population survey, no fewer than 63 per cent had severe chronic physical health problems. Turning to adverse physical health events during the preceding year, only 6 per cent of normal subjects reported such an event, whereas 28 per cent of depressed subjects had experienced a major setback in their health. Depressed subjects of course complain more about their physical health than normal subjects even when there are no objective signs of organic physical disease, so the judgements in this study were made on objective evidence where possible and not simply on the subjects' opinions of their health.

One of the most interesting findings of this study was that depressed elderly subjects with severe chronic ill health were less likely to be receiving specialist treatment for depression than their counterparts in good physical health. The author speculated that the GPs understood and sympathised with depressed mood in physically ill patients and did not feel it appropriate or necessary to treat the depression on its own merit.

Prevention of physical illness and alleviation of accompanying handicaps might make a substantial impact on the occurrence of depression in the elderly. It is particularly tempting to hope that measures aimed at reducing the prevalence of cerebrovascular disease in middle-aged and elderly people may lead to a reduction in the severer forms of depression. However, the wide range of illnesses found in depression suggests that physical illness acts largely through its meaning for the individual rather than through biological mechanisms. A loss of mobility so often requires the sufferer to become more dependent on others to maintain social relationships. The implications of imminent future mortality of a stroke or heart attack are known to everyone. It is likely that the anxiety provoked by serious illness compounded by the irritation and frustration of chronic pain or handicap predispose to depression in the susceptible individual.

The sensitive management of elderly patients with physical illness by the primary care team opens up the possibility of preventive mental health work in a variety of ways. Firstly, considerable improvements in the quality of life can be made by the provision of appropriate aids in the home to assist with tasks of daily living. Domiciliary occupational therapists and physiotherapists give specialist advice on such aids and also give guidance on appropriate furniture, mobility aids and special clothing. More traditionally, district nurses and care attendants considerably lighten the load of a family caring for a sick person by providing a 'getting up' and 'putting to bed' service, regular baths and supervision of medication.

Physically ill patients hate being a burden to their relatives, and the patients' morale can be lifted by the provision of help to the carers. Simply offering practical help may be enough to prevent a loss of morale. However, it is also possible that there is a role for someone to talk over the implications of the illness or handicap with the patients and their families. Some diseases having frightening connotations: 'stroke', 'coronary', 'diabetes' and 'cancer' are words that may have devastating implications for the patient which may be quite inaccurate. It is this author's personal view that good nurses and remedial therapists do explore these issues with patients in the course of their daily work, and that 'psychological help' is very often more acceptable when provided at the same time as practical assistance. Perhaps more time should be spent in training therapists to 'talk as they work'.

The main role of the GP is to initiate an effective scheme of management and to coordinate the input of the other health and social services professionals.

Psychosocial causes

What of the impact of other losses? Sadness is the natural response to loss and, in the lay person's view, depression is caused by unfortunate circumstances and insuperable problems. Depressed patients therefore naturally seek to understand their illness by discovering reasonable explanations in terms of the events of their lives. Old age is a time of loss, of bereavement of family and friends, of loss of income and status with retirement and of loss of health. As a group, elderly people are poorer financially and more likely to be living alone and in poor housing than any other age group. Even so, psychiatrists have been reluctant to view these social changes as anything other than 'triggers', firing off a depression in a previously susceptible person who would sooner or later develop depression anyway.

Recent research findings demonstrating biological changes in depressed patients and the good response of depression to appropriate medication have emphasised the organic, biological side of the problem, and little emphasis has been give to the impact of social change and psychological distress. However, in the past fifteen years there have been several studies demonstrating that depressed patients experience more severely adverse life events of all kinds before the onset of depression. (Paykel et al, 1969; Brown et al, 1973). Brown and his team at Bedford College, London, have taken the argument further and have suggested that all depression is primarily caused by psychosocial factors. The evidence that this is the cause in the vast majority of minor episodes of depression in younger people is striking, and this evidence is eloquently and convincingly presented in Brown and Harris's book *The Social Origins of Depression* (1978). But what of depression in old age?

Murphy's study used Brown's method to compare the rates of life events in the year before onset in 100 elderly depressed subjects and in a group of 168 normal elderly. The same period of one year before interview was also used in the case of normal subjects. Depression in old age was found to be closely associated with adversity. Events involving loss, such as bereavement, separation and so on, were implicated just as in younger subjects. Often the loss was irretrievable; the older we are, the less we can expect to reverse the circumstances which arise as the outcome of severe events.

Severe events of certain kinds — financial loss, forced change of residence, family trouble with police, adverse health events — were related to social class. In general, the more prosperous social classes are protected from a good many adverse experiences. Take for example the situation of an only son moving away from home to take up a new job, leaving his widowed elderly mother living alone. A middle-class mother will often have the savings, the social expertise and the previous experience of travel to give her the opportunity of travelling to see him frequently. Her son will have a car to visit her in between times and he will keep in touch by phone every week. On the other hand, a poorer working-class son may find it extremely difficult and time-consuming to visit by public transport, his mother will not be in the habit of negotiating long distances alone and she may not have a phone. I would suggest that the significance of the move for the working-class older woman is more likely to be adverse. Furthermore, in Murphy's study there was often a background of social disadvantage in the depressed subjects. Major housing problems and financial hardship, for example, were commonplace, although rarely complained about by the subjects directly.

Murphy's survey of community elderly showed a higher prevalence of depression in working-class subjects compared with middle-class elderly. Lowenthal (1964) also found an association between low socioeconomic status and psychiatric symptoms in the elderly in the general population. However, Weissman and Myers found no raised prevalence of depression in lower socioeconomic groups. The explanation for these diverse results may be that many severely adverse events are not class-related — bereavement and illness involving close family members, for example, occur in all social classes.

It might be thought that the milder 'reactive' or 'neurotic' depressions are most likely to follow adverse life events, but this is not the case, and in Murphy's study similar proportions of 'neurotic' depressions and 'psychotic' depressions followed severe life events. Post (1972) also commented on the apparently 'reactive' nature of many of the classic psychotic depressions, pointing out the misuse of the term 'endogenous' as applied to severe depression where physiological symptoms predominate.

Having said that poor physical health and adverse social circumstances precede the onset of depression, it is also clear that the majority of elderly people remain remarkably cheerful. It is only those who are vulnerable in some way that react to adverse circumstances with depression. Lowenthal (1965) demonstrated that the presence of an intimate confidant was associated with good morale and positive mental health. Further, she showed that it is not those who are lifelong isolates by choice who adapt badly to old age stesses, but those who had tried to establish good relationships, sought the intimacy of others but had failed to establish an intimate tie, who were most at risk. Those who had previously had a good relationship but were now without one fared relatively better. These findings were borne out by Murphy's community study in which 30 per cent of elderly subjects who reported a lack of a confiding relationship were found to be depressed. Conversely, 39 per cent of depressed patients attending psychiatric treatment reported a lack of confidant. Two-thirds of those without a confidant reported that they had never had a confiding relationship.

It seems likely that self-reports of intimacy in relationships are largely a reflection of the subject's capacity for intimacy, that is, the personality of the individual. This was borne out in that seemingly distant social support offered by a child or brother or sister, sometimes living many miles from the subject, perceived as 'close' and appeared to protect against depression. The key to these seemingly distant social supports was the feeling of reciprocal warmth, trust and a sense of being valued that they engendered.

It is hard to judge the relevance of findings about the importance of psychosocial factors to the primary prevention of depression. An improvement in the financial status of the elderly would certainly reduce the frequency of some class-related events. Financial security brings with it a sense of control over options for the future. The ability to choose whether to move house, whether to take a holiday, whether to employ private domestic help in the home — all these are real options for a middle-class property-owning elderly person, disabled or not. A sense of mastery over future options is one component of hope, and it is the possibility of renewal of hope that prevents depression from becoming chronic.

The question remains whether it is possible to provide alternative effective social supports for those with no close relatives but who retain the capacity for making close ties. Day centres for elderly people, luncheon clubs and the many hundreds of informal clubs all exist to foster supportive relationships and, it is anticipated, improve general morale. The popularity of these clubs suggests that they do indeed provide a good deal of friendship and a sense of 'belonging' for those who attend regularly. Whether or not such clubs can provide sufficient support to prevent depression in those faced with a severe adverse life event obviously depends on the quality of the relationships established.

If we take at face value the finding that approximately a third of elderly people who lack a confiding relationship report that at some time in their lives they felt close to someone, there is surely the possiblity of stretching that capacity for intimacy and establishing a supportive relationship. However, the provision of formal clubs and social gatherings is probably of less importance than the overall social environment of a neighbourhood. Coordinated planning of housing and social services and thoughtful development by town planners can have a vital impact on the social life of the elderly. The provision of cheap and convenient transport, architectural schemes which encourage neighbours to meet, the provision of local food markets which provide a focus for daily activity — these may well be more preventive of social isolation than the hopeful provision of residents' lounges in sheltered housing schemes and special clubs, both of which tend to be patronised by the habitual extrovert.

An alternative approach to prevention of depression is to tackle the immediate precipitating cause — the seriously adverse life event. Life events are after all the stuff of life — bereavement, separations, illness occur to all of us at some stage of our lives. It has been suggested that intervention by prophylactic counselling after an event has occurred may reduce distress and thereby prevent depression developing in vulnerable individuals. Bereavement counselling schemes have been started on just such tenets of faith. 'Counselling' is an unfortunate term — it smacks of a patronising notion that the client is being given advice from those who know best what is good for him. What these schemes actually offer is a person to act as a listener and supportive befriender in a time of crisis. Many bereaved elderly are surrounded by concerned and caring relatives and friends who provide all the support needed; however, about a third of the very elderly have no living relatives left, and grief must often be borne alone.

The most difficult period for the bereaved is the few weeks after the funeral. The immediate shock of a death is attenuated by a natural protective feeling of numbness and the business of arranging the administrative details consequent upon a bereavement. But once the children have returned to their own homes and the neighbours have retreated a little, the elderly are often left isolated and unvisited. Their own family doctors who may be the most acceptable visitors are frequently neglectful. In one major study, two-thirds of elderly widows had not received a visit from their doctor in the six months after bereavement (Bowling & Cartwright, 1982).

Age Concern, a voluntary organisation promoting the welfare of elderly people in Great Britain, has set up a number of bereavement counselling schemes and closely monitored their development and problems (Barker, 1983). The aim has been to provide a well-matched local volunteer, trained by professionals in the problems of the bereaved, to act as listener and confidant over the months or, if necessary, years after a bereavement. The major problem has been to attract the right clients — those most at risk who could benefit from the service. Professionals are slow to make use of the service and do not always refer appropriately.

The question remains as to whether those who are willing to be 'counselled' are the ones at risk of developing depressive illness. Subjects accepting such a service have already recognised their need to talk of their bereavement and believe in the value of support from others in a crisis. It is those who are ill at ease in interpersonal discussion who may be most at risk of breakdown and yet are likeliest to refuse help. The Age Concern counselling scheme, and similar schemes in Europe and the US, do not claim to prevent depressive illness, but rather seek to offer a support service to all in need, thus providing very real support to the distressed. However, it is unlikely that they have an important role in the reduction of the incidence of true depressive illness.

More valuable perhaps would be an improvement of primary health care. Greater attention to the physical health and mobility of elderly people as mentioned above and more active intervention by GPs at an earlier stage of disability may by one of the few practical measures which will reduce the numbers of depressed elderly

In conclusion, current knowledge of the causes of depression suggests that there are no known primary measures of prevention which are, realistically, likely to be effective on their own. A general raising of living standards in the elderly population and an improvement in health care services are the two major changes which at present offer the greatest hope of prevention.

SECONDARY PREVENTION

While the psychiatric training of GPs during their undergraduate years has improved enormously in the last two decades, sadly this training normally still takes place in psychiatric hospitals and teaching hospital psychiatric units where students are unlikely to meet the sort of depressed elderly patients encountered in general practice. The early identification of cases and appropriate treatment by GPs requires a raising of their vigilance and an anticipatory approach to those at greatest risk.

This chapter has already discussed the large untapped pool of 'unrecognised' depression. On the whole, these depressions are at the milder end of the spectrum. However, a good deal of controversy surrounds the question of whether the majority of patients with depression in the community can be treated effectively by medical or other means. Recently, however, there has been renewed interest in a technique known as 'cognitive therapy', a brief structured psychotherapy derived partly from dynamic psychotherapy and partly from behaviour therapy. Cognitive therapy for depression is founded on the idea that abnormality of mood is a consequence of primary abnormalities of cognition, that is in judging, reasoning and remembering. A depressed person may have irrational beliefs about himself and his worthlessness, may make arbitrary incorrect assumptions about himself and those around him.

Early clinical trials with younger patients with mild depressions were promising (Rush, 1977), and cognitive therapy was shown to be marginally more effective than tricyclic antidepressants in a trial by Blackburn and his colleagues (1981). Encouraging results have recently been decribed with older depressed patients (Gallagher & Thompson, 1983). It is very early to draw any conclusions about the efficacy of cognitive therapy without a far greater number of clinical trials, and there remains the practical issue of who would acquire the technical skills and offer a service to patients in general practice if it does prove to be a useful treatment. One hope is that it could lead to a more rational approach to the prescribing of antidepressant drugs, since it would offer a constructive alternative in the family doctor's treatment options.

PREVENTION OF HANDICAP IN DEPRESSION

The natural history of severe depression in old age is unknown. The expansion of the elderly population has coincided with pharmaceutical advances in the treatment of depression and the widespread use of ECT for major depressive illness. The recognition of the treatability of depression at all ages ensures that, once depression is diagnosed, the patient will almost certainly receive some form of active treatment, usually psychotropic medication. One of the major problems of this willingness to prescribe psychotropic drugs is that patients often receive drugs over a prolonged period of months and years, often far beyond the need for medication. Both in general practice and in hospital outpatients there is a need for more regular review of medication than is generally carried out. If relapse occurs following withdrawal of medication, it is an easy matter to institute treatment again if patients are kept under surveillance. In spite of advances in physical treatments, outcome studies suggest that, over a prolonged period, depression in old age pursues a relapsing, chronic course in the majority of cases. It is probable that currently used regimes of treatment do not prevent relapse or discourage the development of chronic social impairment.

Post (1972) published two major follow-up studies of patients treated at the Maudsley Hospital: a group of 81 patients first seen in 1950 and followed up for six years and, secondly, a group of 92 patients treated in the 1960s following the introduction of tricyclic antidepressants. Results were remarkably similar for the two cohorts. Over the course of three years, rather less than a third made a lasting recovery. Murphy's one-year follow-up of 124 patients, of whom only a third were inpatients, showed similar findings. The study was carried out in three London boroughs in East London, where comprehensive services existed for the elderly, and very few elderly patients would have been referred elsewhere. Only a third had recovered by the end of the first year, a third had an apparently favourable response to treatment but had relapsed, and the remaining third were either dead (14 per cent) or chronically depressed and suffering from considerable social impairment as a result of their illness.

The most important prognostic indicators were, firstly, the initial severity of the illness and, secondly, continuing poor physical health. Patients who had severe psychotic depression had the worst outcome: only 10 per cent had recovered by the end of the year.

The third prognostic factor of major significance was severe life events occurring during the follow-up year. Events were only included if they were independent, in the sense that they could not have come about as a result of the depression itself. Events such as bereavement and major setbacks in the health of close family members were much commoner in the poor-outcome group.

Disappointingly, the presence of a supportive close relationship did not appear to influence outcome once depression had become establised. Since much social management and treatment, for example in day hospitals, is justified by the theoretical advantages of providing supportive alternative social relationships for those who lack them, the question arises whether these social methods are effective. Since a close supportive relationship or intimate confidant has been shown to be important in protecting mentally healthy older people from developing depression in the face of adversity, why is this protective function lost once depression has become established? The reason may be that severe depression interferes with the capacity to engage in mutual interpersonal relationships — the depressed patient is self-preoccupied, withdrawn and unable to feel close to others. Thus depression itself socially isolates the patient and interferes with the healing effect of close relationships with others.

All the outcome studies of depression in old age have been carried out on the more severely disturbed patients referred to specialist psychiatric services. Since patients with less severe illnesses appear (as discussed earlier) to have a better prognosis, there are grounds for being rather more optimistic about mildly ill patients if they are properly treated in general practice.

It is now customary to treat depressed younger patients with prophylactic medication for many months after an episode, with the hope of preventing relapse. The patient with recurrent depression is now usually advised to take continuous medication, either tricyclic antidepressant medication or lithium carbonate. There are a number of studies suggesting that patients with recurrent depression taking prophylactic medication have fewer depressive episodes and are less likely to require hospital treatment.

However, studies of prophylaxis in depression are notable for their exclusion of elderly people. A search of the literature during the preparation of this chapter revealed no published studies of prophylactic antidepressant medication in the elderly or lithium prophylaxis in the elderly. Such studies are urgently needed. Drugs used to treat depression give rise to particular problems in elderly people, and if we are to prescribe such drugs over long periods, there needs to be good evidence of their efficacy.

Tricyclic antidepressants are, on the whole, sedative and produce postural hypotension. Side-effects such as dry mouth, constipation and dizziness may not be tolerated by the elderly. Futhermore, plasma levels are difficult to predict for a given dose, and close monitoring of dosage by clinical interview is difficult to achieve outside the hospital setting. Special care is needed in patients with cardiovascular and renal disease.

Newer antidepressants which carry a reduced risk of side-effects and are generally less hazardous to prescribe, such as mianserin, trazodone and nomifensine, are as yet of unproven efficacy in old-age depression. Lithium also carries high risks in elderly patients, particularly those with impaired renal function. The supervision of plasma levels by regular blood testing can prove quite difficult in patients without their own transport. Elderly patients on lithium seem especially prone to develop tremor, excessive weight gain and diminished thyroid function. This is probably because these unwanted effects are dose-related and elderly patients should be maintained at the lower end of the therapeutic range. Thyroid and renal functions should be monitored more frequently than in younger patients.

The sad fact remains that in current clinical practice a good deal of effort must be directed towards minimising the social handicaps of patients with continuing chronic depressive illness. The major aim is to help the patient and her (or his) family to lead as normal a life as possible, given her special disabilities. Day care facilities, whether day hospitals run by health service professionals or day centres run by social services or voluntary agencies, provide diversion for the self-preoccupied and a convenient way for professionals to detect relapse and remission. They also play a valuable role in relieving a caring relative of a few hours' contact with a permanently gloomy elderly person living in the house.

The patient and her family may also be helped by regular support from a professional worker such as a visiting community nurse, social worker or doctor, but at present the role of supportive psychotherapy of this kind in maintaining hope in the chronically depressed elderly patient is unknown.

SUMMARY OF PREVENTATIVE MEASURES IN DEPRESSION IN OLD AGE

Strategies for primary prevention

1. Improvement of the financial and consequently the social status of elderly people.
2. a. Improvement in the provision of health care services, with the hope of early detection and treatment of physical illness.
   b. Education of medical students about illness in the elderly.
   c. Provision of easily accessible primary care services.
3. Research into biological factors likely to be aetiologically important in severe depressive psychoses.
4. The provision of alternative social supports for elderly people who are living alone and have lost their major supportive relationships by the provision of day care facilities, clubs, voluntary visitors.

Strategies for prevention of handicap in depression

1. The education of GPs as to early detection and treatment of depression by social, psychological and medical means.
2. The encouragement of research into the efficacy of prophylactic drug regimes.
3. The provision of social support to patients and relatives via day centres, day hospitals, visiting community psychiatric nurses and other professional workers.
4. The giving of special attention to the maintenance of physical health and nutrition of sufferers.

SUICIDE

Epidemiology

Suicide rates are higher for elderly people than for any other age group. The rate for elderly men over 65 years is approximately 20 per 1 000 000 in the United Kingdom. This represents a rate three times as high as that for men between 15 and 24 years old. The rate is substantially lower in women throughout life, reaching a peak of about 11 per 100 000 in middle age and remaining at this level throughout the sixties, seventies and eighties (Mortality Statistics, 1977). The pattern in the United States is very similar.

Interestingly, the suicide rate for men has dropped dramatically since the early 1960s. In 1961 the UK rate for male suicides over 65 years of age was 35 per 100 000. In Britain this decline has been traditionally attributed to the change of domestic gas from coal gas to the less noxious natural gas. However, similar trends downwards in elderly suicides have not been seen in the Netherlands where a similar change in domestic gas took place rather earlier. Furthermore, an even steeper decline in elderly male suicide rates has been noted over the same period in the United States where other suicide methods, principally shooting, have been traditionally more popular and where gas supply has remained unchanged (Resnik & Cantor, 1970). Recent studies in Alberta, Canada, have confirmed that rates in elderly men have dropped, but cohort studies suggest that each generation seems to maintain a fairly stable suicide rate throughout life (Hellon & Solomon, 1980). As noted earlier in this chapter, sucide rates are rising amoung young people. This cohort effect may lead to an upswing of elderly suicides in another half century.

Suicide statistics are notoriously inaccurate, erring on the low side. This may be particularly true for physically ill elderly people, where death by overdose of drugs is all too easily ascribed to accidental error. Relatives rarely inform the Coroner of a suicide victim's depressed mood unless specifically asked and, surprisingly, often they are not asked. Also, the distress caused to families by the suicide of a relative is so great there is a natural tendency, where a measure of doubt exists, to ascribe a death to any cause other than suicide.

On the whole, elderly people who attempt suicide intend to kill themselves and use serious means. Elderly men in Britain frequently hang themselves, use car exhaust fumes or suffocate themselves with polythene bags, and American men use firearms. The majority of women, however, choose overdose by drugs, or poison. The fatal intent of elderly suicide attempts is in marked contrast to younger people, where the majority of attempts fall into the 'parasuicide' category, where intent is less clearly formulated and the attempt is a way of registering distress. Failed suicide attempts in the elderly are usually 'bungled' jobs and the risk of future suicide remains high. Kreitman (1976) found that 8 per cent of older males who survived a suicide attempt later killed themselves.

Unfortunately there is a tendency in society to consider suicide in old age, but not at any other age, as, somehow, normal. It is commonplace to hear comments that suicide in the old is the rational response to a hopeless, irreversible decline and that suicide should not necessarily by discouraged but accepted as a proper existentialist stance. This view gains credence from the finding that in many studies of suicide and attempted suicide, between 35 and 85 per cent of subjects were suffering from serious physical illness (Sainsbury, 1972; Barraclough, 1971). This argument ignores the findings on the rate of treatable mental illness in those who kill themselves. It also ignores the serious impact that suicide has on the immediate relatives. Suicide is the most potent demonstration of desolation and brings home to the family in the most wounding and frequently catastrophic fashion their inability to console or help someone close to them. The stigma of a parent's suicide can remain for ever on the conscience of the children.

In recent years it has become clear that suicide in the elderly usually occurs with a background of depressive illness. Barraclough's (1971) study of 80 elderly suicides rated 87 per cent suffering from affective disorder, a judgement based on interviews with close relatives and information from medical records. Key symptoms of depression which were recorded for these suicides and which appear to be signs of grave risk were persistent insomnia, weight loss, hypochondriasis, difficulty in concentration, severe anxiety and delusional ideas of guilt and illness. A history of alcohol abuse adds further risk in the elderly, as at all ages. Depressive illness, however, is the key factor for suicide and, as has been noted earlier, depression is very closely associated with physical illness. This is possibly the reason why so many suicides have a history of grave physical illness.

The problem with all studies of completed suicides is that information is necessarily collected retrospectively. Researchers investigating a history of depressive illness may well overestimate the prevalence of depression because relatives may seek to explain a relative's suicide in terms of mental illness. Suicide studies, moreover, include only those subjects where an inquest has reached the verdict of suicide, presumably cases where the Coroner had no doubt in his mind that suicide had occurred. A known history of previous depressive illness is one of the factors which would sway the Coroner's verdict towards suicide. It is possible therefore that the rate of mental illness in those who commit suicide may be overestimated.

Social factors

Living alone and recent bereavement are also important ancillary factors underlying the decision for suicide. The background theme for the decision is a personal sense of desolation and loss. There may be some rational suicides among isolated physically ill elderly who know there will be no improvement in the future, but it is likely that the majority are depressed and that a substantial but important minority have a major depressive psychosis.

The role of the doctor in prevention

Suicide is theoretically preventable. If it is true that a substantial proportion of those who kill themselves have a treatable depressive illness, then early detection and treatment should be effective prevention. Unfortunately, as noted earlier, GPs are reluctant to diagnose depression in the elderly and, even where it is recognised, they are less likely to refer them to psychiatrists than younger patients (Kessel & Shepherd, 1962). Furthermore, suicide victims have normally seen their doctors quite recently: 50 per cent of Barraclough's elderly suicides had seen their GP within the week before the suicide, 90 per cent within the previous three months. They had consulted for physical symptoms, and presumably the doctors had failed to spot the depression lurking behind the reported physical illness.

The opportunities for intervention are potentially much improved if GPs learn to be vigilant with those at risk. Having recognised that an elderly person is depressed, the GP should always enquire about suicidal thoughts and plans. Even if thoughts are fleeting, the doctor should never unwittingly provide an easy means of suicide by prescribing antidepressant drugs to an unsupervised depressed patient with suicidal ideas. Once the doctor has spotted the problem, a speedily available psychiatric service should, ideally, provide that necessary back-up of treatment opportunities.

Crisis intervention and the Samaritans

The Samaritans are a lay organisation in the UK which operates with almost nationwide coverage and provides a telephone advice service to potential suicides. Their work has attracted a good deal of attention and they claim to have prevented suicides. However, the overall rates of suicide among young and middle-aged people who make up the bulk of the 'clients' has not dropped since the Samaritans' service began. Ten years ago, two-thirds of a random sample of people over 65 years had not heard of the Samaritans (Atkinson, 1970) and, although this is probably no longer the case, the Samaritans appear to have made no great headway in reaching the elderly population. A spokesman for the Samaritans has recently estimated that no more than 2 per cent of clients are elderly (Day, 1983). The Samaritans do outstanding work supporting younger adults in times of desperation and crisis, but the users of the service appear to be more closely akin to 'parasuicides' than to those at risk of suicide. Any crisis intervention service aimed at elderly people needs to reach those at risk in their own homes. So far, no such service is provided.

Public health meausres

The easy availability of the means of suicide might be considered a good target for intervention. Hudgens (1983), pointed out that an effective method of preventing suicide is to make it harder to do; no one now jumps off the Empire State Building since the authorities put a fence round the observation platform! Similarly, very few people shoot themselves in the United Kingdom because firearms are not generally available. Again, the numbers of suicides from coal gas poisoning dropped from 1350 in 1967 to 8 in 1977. Quite small changes in policy can have a marked effect on methods used. For example, the decision of a large British chain of retail chemists to stop the sale of aspirin in large containers was a direct consequence of the publicity arising from Kessel's study of self-poisoning among young people and his highlighting of the ease with which large quantities of aspirin could be purchased (Kessel, 1965)

In the United Kingdom, drugs are the main means of suicide in the elderly, especially psychotropic drugs. Barbiturates used to be the main culprits, but this hazard has diminished since benzodiazepines have now replaced them as the most popular prescribed hypnotics. However, tricyclic antidepressants remain lethal. A relatively small dose may kill an elderly person, and tricyclics should never be left with a depressed person living alone who is known to be at risk. An expensive but potentially efficacious method of preventing drugs being consumed on impulse is to prescribe drugs in 'blister packs' where determination to take an overdose has to be maintained over the course of several minutes. This may prove a surprisingly effective 'brake' on the suicidal impulse. Another helpful influence may be the development of antidepressant drugs which are not lethal when taken in large quantities. The efficacy of the newer safer antidepressants is unfortunately unproven at present.

Finally, there is a *role for the Coroner* in the prevention of future suicides. Coroners rarely take an active part in notifying concerned professional workers of a suspected suicide or in encouraging them to attend inquests. The author, when providing a psychiatric service for the elderly in East London, was never invited to the inquest on a patient who was receiving psychiatric treatment from a member of her team. She often learnt only by chance of the suicide from relatives, neighbours or community nurses. Surely doctors would learn more of the risk factors involved if relevant personal cases were brought to their attention?

SUMMARY OF SUICIDE PREVENTION MEASURES

1. The education of GPs to recognise the risk of suicide in depression, especially in men with physical illness, in those living alone and with few social supports.

2. The development of effective crisis intervention services which are able to reach elderly people when they need them.

3. The reduction of the means of suicide available, by firearms control, control of the sale of poisons and drugs, packaging to prevent impulse overdose, cautious prescribing to depressed patients.

4. The development of safe and efficacious antidepressant drugs which are not lethal in overdose.

5. The encouragement of closer liaison between the Coroner and professional workers.

REFERENCES

Atkinson J M 1970 The Samaritans and the elderly. In: Proceedings of the 5th International Cogress for Suicide Prevention. London

Barker J 1983 Volunteer bereavement counselling schemes: a report on a monitoring exercise. Age Concern, London

Barraclough B M 1971 Suicide in the elderly. In: Kay D W K, Walk A (eds) Recent developments in psychogeriatrics. Headley, London

Blackburn I, Bishop S, Glen A I M, Whalley, Christie J E 1981 The efficacy of cognitive therapy in depression. British Journal of Psychiatry 139: 181–189

Blazer D G, Williams C D 1980 The epidemiology of dysphoria and depression in the elderly population. American Journal of Psychiatry 137: 439–444
Bollerup T R 1975 Prevalence of mental illness among 70 year olds domiciled in nine Copenhagen surburbs. The Glostrup survey. Acta Psychiatrica Scandinavica 51: 327–339
Bowling A, Cartwright A 1982 Life after death. Tavistock, London
Brown G W, Harris T O, Peto J 1973 Life events and psychiatric disorder. Part 2. Nature of the causal link. Psychological Medicine 3: 159–76
Brown G W, Harris T O, 1978 Social origins of depression. Tavistock, London
Day G 1983 Personnal communication.
Gallagher D E, Thompson L W 1982 Treatment of major depressive disorder in older adult outpatients with brief psychotherapies. Psychotherapy: Theory, Research and Practice 19: 482–490
Goldberg D, Kay C, Thompson L 1976 Psychiatric morbidity in general practice and the community. Pschological Medicine 6: 565–569
Grauer H 1977 Depression in the aged: theoretical concepts, Journal of the American Geriatrics Society 25: 447–449
Gruer R 1975 Needs of the elderly in the Scottish borders. Scottish Home and Health Department, Edinburgh
Gurland, B J 1976 The comparative frequency of depression in various adult age groups. Journal of Gerontology 31: 283–292
Gurland B, Dean L, Cross P, Golden R 1980 The epidemiology of depression and dementia in the elderly; the use of multiple indicators of these conditions. In: Cole J O, Barrett J E (eds) Psychopathology in the aged. Raven Press, New York
Guze S B, Robins L 1970 Suicide and primary affective disorders. British Journal of Psychiatry. 117: 437–438
Harris, L 1975 The myth and reality of aging in America. The National Council on the Aging. Washington DC
Hendrickson E, Levy R, Post F 1979 Average evoked responses in relation to congnitive and affective state of elderly psychiatric patients. British Journal of Psychiatry 134: 494–501
Hellon C P, Solomon M I 1980 Suicide and age in Alberta, Canada 1951–1977: the changing profile. Archives of General Psychiatry 37: 505–510
Hudgens R 1983 Preventing suicide. Editorial comment. New England Journal of Medicine 308: 897–898
Jacoby R, Dolan R J, Levy R, Baldy R 1983 Quantitative computed tomography in elderly depressed patients. British Journal of Psychiatry 143: 124–127
Jacoby R, Levy R 1980 Computed tomography in the elderly. 3. Affective disorders. British Journal of Psychiatry 136: 270–275
Jolley D J, Arie T 1976 Psychiatric services for the elderly: how many beds. British Journal of Psychiatry 129: 418–423
Kay D W K, Norris V, Post F 1956 Prognosis in psychiatric disorders of the elderly: an attempt to define the indicators of early death and early recovery. Journal of Mental Science 102: 129–140
Kay D W K, Bergmann K 1966 Physical disability and mental health in old age. Journal of Psychosomatic Research 10: 3–12
Kessel N, Shepherd M 1962 Neurosis in hospital and general practice. Journal of Mental Science 108: 159–166
Kessel N 1965 Self-poisoning. British Medical Journal ii: 1265–70 and ii: 1336–40
Klerman G L 1976 Age and clinical depression: today's youth in the twenty-first century. Journal of Gerontology 31: 318–323
Kreitman N 1976 Age and parasuicide 'attempted suicide'. Psychological Medicine 6: 113-121
Leighton A H 1963 The character of danger. Basic Books, New York
Lewis A 1936 Melancholia: prognostic study and case material. Journal of Mental Science 82: 488–558
Lowenthal M F 1964 Social isolation and mental illness in old age. American Sociological Review 29: 54–70
Lowenthal, M F 1965 Antecedents of isolation and mental illness in old age. Archives of General Psychiatry 12: 245–254
Mendlewicz J 1976 The age factor in depressive illness: some genetic considerations. Journal of Gerontology 31: 300–303

Murphy E 1982 Social origins of depression in old age. British Journal of Psychiatry 141: 135–142
Murphy E, Grundy E 1984 A comparative study of bed usage by younger and older depressed patients. Psychological Medicine 14: 445–450
Murphy E 1983 The prognosis of depression in old age. British Journal of Psychiatry 142: 111–119
Murphy G E, Wetzel R D 1980 Suicide risk by birth cohort in the United States 1949 to 1974. Archives of General Psychiatry 37: 519–523
Office of Population Censuses and Surveys 1977 Mortality Statistics. HMSO, London
Paykel E S, Myers J K, Dienelt M N, Klerman G, Lindenthal J J, Pepper M P 1969 Life events and depression: a controlled study. Archives of General Psychiatry 21: 753–760
Post F 1969 The relationship to physical health of the affective illnesses in the elderly. 8th International Congress of Gerontology Proceedings. Washington D C
Post F 1972 The management and nature of depressive illnesses in late life: a follow-through study. British Journal of Psychiatry 121: 393–404
Resnik H L P, Cantor J 1970 Suicide and aging. Journal of the American Geriatrics Society 18: 152-158
Roth M, Kay D W K 1956 Affective disorder arising in the senium II Physical disability as an aetiological factor. Journal of Mental Science 102: 141–150
Rush A J, Beck A T, Kovacs M, Hollon S D 1977 article Cognitive Therapy and Research 1: 410–421
Sainsbury P 1962 Suicide in late life. Gerontologia Clinica 4: 161
Skegg D C G, Doll R, Perry J 1977 Use of medicines in general practice. British Medical Journal i: 1561–1563
Solomon M I, Hellon C P 1980 Suicide and age in Alberta, Canada 1951–1977. Archives of General Psychiatry 37: 511–513
Weissman M M, Myers J K 1978 Affective disorders in a US urban community. Archives of General Psychiatry 35: 1304–1311
Williamson J et al 1964 Old people at home, their unreported needs. Lancet i: 1117–1120

Nutritional aspects of ageing: present status and implications

INTRODUCTION

The role of nutrition in ageing begins with a definition of when ageing occurs. For the purposes of this status report, we consider that ageing begins in the young adult and continues to impair tissue function throughout adult life. The relationship of nutrition to this process can be divided into three sections. First, it has to be determined how far nutrition can influence the progressive deterioration in tissue structure and function as the adult advances in age. Second, nutrition is one of the most likely aetiological factors in age-related degenerative diseases such as atherosclerosis and cancer. Finally, we have very imperfect knowledge about the nutrient needs of people who are old and in general eat less food. The question here is whether the reduced consumption of food by older people results in intakes of nutrients that are insufficient to maintain health and tissue function

In this background report, the current state of knowledge in each of these areas will be reviewed. Then, at the end of each section, the significance of the findings for determining the role of nutrition in public health planning for the elderly will be considered in terms of preventive action throughout adult life.

Mention should be made here of some more extensive reviews of the above topics by Exton-Smith and Caird (1980) who deal with the literature on nutrition and ageing, while supplements to the American Journal of Clinical Nutrition (1979, 1982) describe the conclusions reached by panels of experts about the role of nutrition in the aetiology of chronic disease in the elderly and the evidence for deficiency of certain nutrients among the elderly. Finally, Posner (1979) provides a detailed analysis of the Nutrition Program for Older Americans mandated by the US Congress.

NUTRITION AND THE AGEING PROCESS

Body composition

Body compsition undergoes continuous change in the adult as he or she ages. Lean body mass is represented by the amount of radioactivity from ^{40}K, a natural isotope of potassium which is concentrated in the cells (Forbes & Reina, 1970; Steen et al, 1979). Body content of ^{40}K progressively decreases throughout adult life, while an increase in body fat content compensates for the weight loss, so that body weight remains little affected.

This pattern of change in body composition is not uniformly distributed between tissues. As compared with young adults, men of 70 years have lost about 10 per cent of the weight of their kidneys and lungs, the liver loses 19 per cent, while skeletal muscle diminishes by 40 per cent (Korenchevsky, 1961). This extensive loss of muscle is confirmed by a study using neutron activation in combination with ^{40}K measurements (Cohn et al, 1980) and also by measurement of urinary output of creatinine and of 3-methyl-histidine (Munro & Young, 1978). We do not know whether this loss is affected by nutritional factors. Finally, bone salts undergo a loss in adult life (osteoporosis) which can lead to facture. The relationship of osteoporosis to calcium and other dietary constituents is discussed later.

Tissue function and metabolism

Throughout adult life, there is a continuous loss in the functional capacity of many tissues and organs. Shock (1971) reports cross-sectional studies of men between the ages of 30 and 80 years. Various physiological functions, including cardiac capacity, maximum capacity for work output, etc., showed decreased function, the rate of loss varying from 20 per cent for nerve velocity to 50 per cent for renal blood flow over the period studied. In addition to the systems reported by Shock, there is a marked decline in the functions of other systems. For example, there is reduced cellular immunity (Callard, 1977). It has been well established that immune mechanisms are also affected by nutrition, but the extent to which improved nutrition can alleviate this age-dependent decline remains unknown.

Metabolic functions are also affected by ageing. Basal energy metabolism decreases by 20 per cent between 30 and 90 years of age, and parallels the reduction in lean body mass (Gregerman, 1967). Because of the reduced lean body mass, turnover of body protein also diminishes with ageing when expressed per unit of body weight (Uauy et al, 1978). Ageing also decreases the capacity of the body to metabolise glucose (Silverstone et al, 1957) and lipids (Kritchevsky, 1979). The latter may be a factor in their progressive accumulation in some tissues. We (Gersovitz et al, 1980) have shown that synthesis of albumin by elderly people is less responsive when dietary protein intake is raised from low to adequate levels. This may imply that synthesis of this secreted protein by older people may be less capable of responding to improved intake of protein. Such a change may account for the reduction in plasma albumin level in older people.

Animal models of nutrition and ageing

Experiments on ageing animals provide our best evidence that the ageing process may be susceptible to nutritional modification. McCay et al (1939) first showed that giving restricted amounts of food to rodents from early life causes them to live longer than do those eating *ad libitum*, an observation that has been repeatedly confirmed. Since the wild rat does not eat *ad libitum*, these experiments may be interpreted to mean that the caged rat on an unlimited intake of food may be undergoing a reduced lifespan that is corrected by restricting food intake and increasing exercise. This parallels the human situation, where excessive intake of food and lack of exercise create an unfavourable environment for optimal survival. In addition to changes in lifespan, the rat fed *ad libitum* shows degenerative changes in tissue function, such as ageing of collagen (Everitt, 1971), neuromuscular paralysis (Everitt et al, 1980) and defective responses of the immunological system (Weindruch et al, 1979) as compared with rats given less food.

In summary, we can conclude that there is compelling evidence of the inexorable change in body composition, tissue function and metabolism throughout adult life. In the case of loss of skeletal density (osteoporosis), there is reason to believe (see later) that both hormonal and nutritional factors can determine the extent of this loss in humans, thus leading to the conclusion that nutrition is worth exploring as a component of the ageing process in tissue function. This conclusion is supported by animal studies. It would thus appear that the effects of the levels of intake of various nutrients on long-term health and preservation of tissue function should be evaluated in conjunction with other determinants of continuing health in the adult, such as exercise. In this respect, the degree of preservation of tissue function during ageing in under-developed countries could provide useful clues regarding the role of individual nutrients in retarding the age-related loss of function. Since the lifestyle and physical work pattern differs in these locations, the role of nutrition in combination with the other factors can perhaps be evaluated more persuasively.

ROLE OF NUTRITION IN AGE-RELATED CHRONIC DISEASES

Evidence from human and animal studies

The role of diet as a factor in the causation of chronic age-related diseases has been much discussed. The evidence relating specific nutrients to these degenerative conditions has been extensively reviewed by a task force in 1978 (American Journal of Clinical Nutrition, 1978). The consensus statements of the panel were less than unanimous but reach the cautious conclusion that intake of fat is related to the process of atherosclerosis, while high salt intakes are related to hypertension. The role of nutrition in the epidemiology of ischaemic heart disease has been reviewed by Oliver (1981). He also concludes cautiously that there is a correlation between incidence of coronary heart disease and diet, fat being the most likely major contributor. Oliver (1981) suggests that intake of essential fatty acids (related to polyunsaturated fatty acid metabolism) may be the most important dietary component in the genesis of atherosclerotic heart disease. The requirements for the essential fatty acid component of fats are small. Ensuring by supplementation that the diet contains enough of these is suggested by him as a practical solution.

The relationship of dietary patterns to cancer incidence has also been extensively explored in animals experimentally and in humans by means of epidemiological studies. A summary of the evidence is provided by Shils (1980), and a recent committee report (Diet, Nutrition and Cancer Committee, 1982) has appeared, evaluating the evidence relating diet and nutrition to the occurence of cancer. In rats, prolonged restriction of energy intake reduces tumour incidence, while reduction in protein intake changes the spectrum of tumours (see review by Guigoz & Munro, 1985). The epidemiological evidence also suggests a relationship between diet and the incidence of cancer. For example, Japanese emigrating to Hawaii lose some of the high incidence of gastric cancer observed in Japan, but achieve the high American frequency of cancer of the large intestine, the effect of environment being evident within ten years. Both fat and dietary fibre are suggested as causal dietary factors.

In spite of much controversy about the role of long-term nutrition in the genesis of age-related degerative disease, it remains uncertain how much the incidence of these conditions in the developed countries is influenced by the long-term eating patterns of the population in conjunction with other factors in lifestyle. The under-developed countries relate to this conclusion in two ways. First, the patterns of degenerative diseases seen in under-developed population could help to provide more conclusive evidence of the role of nutrition and of specific nutrients in the production of such diseases. Second, awareness of the penalties of certain dietary habits as developing countries become more prosperous may help them to avoid the high incidence of the degenerative diseases seen in affluent countries.

NUTRIENT NEEDS AND NUTRITIONAL STATUS OF THE ELDERLY

Dietary allowances and actual nutrient intakes

Allowances for all essential nutrients are provided in the US by the Recommended Dietary Allowances (1980) and similar publications in other countries. Since information about the nutrient needs of adults is mainly based on data gathered on young adults, allowances for older adults are commonly estimated by extrapolation. In the case of the US Recommended Dietary Allowances (RDA), there are only two age categories for adults, namely 23–50 years inclusive, and over 50 years of age. The latter covers a period of continuous change and is palpably inadequate to be representative over such a long period of adult life. Consideration of some major nutrients will show the importance of establishing reliable allowances for the elderly, not to mention the middle-aged (Munro, 1984).

The effect of ageing on energy needs has been explored by a number of investigators. An extensive cross-sectional study was made twenty years ago on American male executives ranging from 20 to 93 years of age who were examined at the Gerontology Center at Baltimore, and who were certainly not representative of the average American population (McGandy et al, 1966). The mean energy intakes of this group declined progressively from 2700 kcal/day at age 30 to 2100 kcal at 80 years of age (Fig. 11.1). This decline was partly accounted for by a reduction over this age-span in basal energy metabolism (200 kcal) in parallel with the decline in lean body mass, whereas the major cause of the reduction in energy expenditures (400 kcal) could be assigned to a larger decline in energy used for physical activity (Fig. 11.1).

Data collected on young and old men and women in Scotland (Munro, 1964a) supports this picture. At age 20 years, male clerks averaged energy

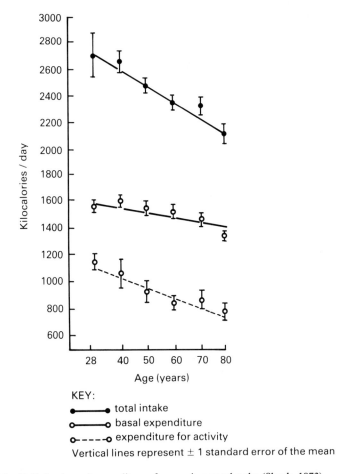

Fig. 11.1 Daily intake and expenditure of energy in normal males (Shock, 1972)

intakes of 3000 kcal per day, whereas clerks at age 50 years consumed 2400 kcal, while retired elderly men averaged 2050 kcal per day. In later life, there is evidence that the rate of reduction in energy intake accelerates. Exton-Smith (1977) studied the same subjects at 70 and at 80 years of age; during the course of this ten-year period, energy intake fell 19 per cent. The most important cause of the accelerated reduction in energy intake was attributed to increasing disabilities limiting the physical activity of the ageing person. This conclusion also applies to nursing-home patients, who commonly show extensive immobility. In the case of a study of nursing homes in Colorado, it was reported by Stiedemann et al (1978) that men averaged 1720 kcal/day and women 1330 kcal intake per day, barely above the energy needs for basal metabolism. The benefits of mobility are illustrated by a comparison of elderly women living in French towns and in the countryside; Debry et al (1980) found that energy intake was appreciably higher among the country-women, presumably because they led more active lives.

One obvious result of the reduction in energy intake accompanying ageing is that other nutrients in the total food intake are liable to be consumed in smaller amounts. In the case of the Baltimore study (McGandy et al, 1966) shown in Figure 12.1, only slight decreases in intakes of iron, thiamin, riboflavin and niacin were observed, and no significant reduction in intake of calcium, vitamin A and ascorbate was seen as age increased. These subjects were better able financially to select foods with good nutritive properties, whereas less privileged groups would not necessarily fare so well. Thus, the low income groups of elderly examined in the Ten-State Survey (1972) had unsatisfactory intakes of certain nutrients. In the case of the women in nursing homes in Colorado studied by Stiedemann et al (1978), average intakes of thiamin, calcium and iron were less than the RDA. Exton-Smith and Stanton (1965) studies old people over the decade 70 to 80 years of age and observed that intakes of all nutrients underwent extensive reduction. Since we largely lack information on the needs of the elderly for individual nutrients, it is not possible to say whether these reduced intakes of nutrients fell below requirements.

The ultimate criterion for requirements must eventually relate to bodily function. Some of the problems associated with using such a criterion for determining adequacy of intake by the elderly is illustrated by the need for ascorbic acid. An intake of 60 mg per day is suggested for adults of all ages (Recommended Dietary Allowances, 1980), while the elderly men in the Baltimore study averaged intakes of much more than this. However, this was a privileged group. In the Ten-State Survey of older US citizens (1972), much lower intakes were reported, and plasma levels of ascorbic acid were unacceptably low for 10 per cent. An interesting study of white blood cell ascorbic acid was carried out on nursing-home cases in Britain (Andrews et al, 1969). The values found were half those obtained in young adults, and the nursing-home diet had to be supplemented with 80 mg ascorbic acid in order to achieve the white cell levels of the young group, indicating that either absorption or intracellular retention of ascorbic acid is less efficient in older people. There was, however, no obvious clinical benefit when, in another study (Burr et al, 1975), nursing-home cases were given supplementary ascorbic acid over a two-year period.

The most extensively studied relationship between diet and changes in body composition with age relate to bone density, which is discussed in detail elsewhere in this volume. Although the process of osteoporosis is generally thought to begin after the age of 40 years (Garn, 1978), Riggs et al (1982) consider that changes are already evident in certain bones after 20 years of age. Men lose bone density more slowly than do women, some of whom experience specially rapid changes following the menopause. The timing and pattern of osteoporotic fracture is thus different in the two sexes. The nutrients most likely to be involved in age-related bone loss are calcium, phosphorus, vitamin D and protein.

The roles of calcium and vitamin D have recently been evaluated by panels of experts (Heaney et al, 1982; Parfitt et al, 1982). Evidence from Yugoslav populations subsisting on local diets either low in calcium or high in calcium (Matkovic et al, 1979) suggests that a major benefit of a high intake from natural sources is to ensure adequate deposition of mineral salts in bone in late adolescence and early adult life. Thereafter bone density declined at the same rate in both Yugoslav populations, but those living in the low-calcium district reached a critical degree of thinness for susceptibility to fracture sooner because of their less dense bones as young adults. There is, however, evidence from studies in both the US and Britain that postmenopausal bone loss can be prevented by intakes of 1.5 g calcium per day (Horsman et al, 1977; Recker et al, 1977; Heaney et al, 1978), or by lower doses (1 g) if oestrogens are also administered (Horsman et al, 1983). The latter is thus similar to the calcium requirement for premenopausal women (Heaney et al, 1978). These levels of calcium intake are much higher than those customarily consumed in the US by middle-aged and elderly women (Heaney et al, 1982), few of whom reach intakes approaching the Recommended Dietary Allowance for calcium of 800 mg per day.

Other dietary factory have been implicated in the occurrence of osteoporosis. Experiments with formula diets (Anand & Linkswiler, 1976) showed that raising only protein intake caused increased loss of calcium in the urine and a negative calcium balance, but Spencer et al (1978) claim that natural sources of protein (e.g. meat) contain enough phosphate to counteract this effect, though Heaney and Recker (1982) conclude that the action of phosphorus is insufficient to compensate significantly for the effects of high intakes of protein. The importance of vitamin D in bone disease in the elderly remains controversial. Deficiency of the vitamin causes osteomalacia, commoner in the elderly in Europe than in the US, where fortification of milk and margarine with vitamin D_2 and more frequent exposure to the ultraviolet rays of sunsine assure a better supply of this vitamin (Parfitt et al, 1982). In recent years, more emphasis has been placed on exercise as a factor in maintaining bone strength. Marathon runners have more dense bones (Aloia et al, 1978a) and it has been found that loss of bone mass in middle-aged women (Aloia et al, 1978b; Krølner et al, 1983) and even in elderly women (Smith et al, 1981) can be halted by exercise over a period of months or years.

Although anaemia due to iron deficiency occurs in certain groups in every country, it is not a major problem among elderly people in developed countries. Even women who have low stores of iron during their reproductive years start to show an increase after the age of 50 years, while men show a progressive increase in stored iron throughout adult life. Nevertheless, the US Ten-State Survey (1972) and of a survey of elderly in Syracuse, New York (Dibble et al, 1967), indicated that the iron intakes of elderly women were often below the Recommended Dietary Allowance of 10 mg per day.

An area of controversy is the protein needs of the elderly. Protein intake falls in parallel with energy intake among the ageing (Munro, 1964a). Protein requirements are often determined by gradually increasing the protein content of the diet from a low level until nitrogen intake and output are equal. Three such nitrogen balance studies have recently been reported on elderly people. In one study (Cheng et al, 1978) young and old prison inmates were fed the same three levels of dietary protein and showed similar responses of nitrogen balance, suggesting similar protein needs. In this study, however, both young and old men received the same energy intakes, although Figure 11.1 shows that elderly men need less energy. Since energy intakes in excess of requirement improve nitrogen balance (Munro, 1964b), the elderly men would probably have required more dietary protein if their energy intake had been appropriate for their diminished needs. The second study was made by Zanni et al (1979) on elderly men who had followed a diet low in protein; the latter causes subjects to retain dietary protein more efficiently and thus does not adequatley reflect the requirements of these elderly adults. Finally, we (Gersovitz et al, 1982) have recently made a month-long study of the nitrogen balances of elderly men and women receiving the recommended adult allowance (0.8 g protein/kg body weight) along with energy intakes appropriate for their need; this level of dietary protein proved to be inadequate as an allowance for some old people, especially the women in the group studied. It seems probable that the elderly need more protein in conjunction with their reduced caloric intakes (Fig. 11.1). A greater need for protein by older people is supported by the higher frequency of illnesses among old people which cause transient losses of body protein requiring replacement from dietary sources.

The nutritional status of elderly populations

In order to determine whether elderly people suffer from nutrient deficiencies, clinical examination and biochemical indices should be used as well as the dietary history. Using these approaches, the British government has made periodic surveys of representative samples of elderly people (Department of Health and Social Security, 1979). These have demonstrated that malnutrition was present in 6 percent of men and 5 per cent of women between 70 and 80 years, and in 12 per cent of men and 8 per cent of women over that age. The most frequent deficiencies seen were protein–calorie malnutrition and (surprisingly) iron deficiency, while intakes of iron, vitamin B_1, folate, vitamin C and vitamin D were judged to be inadequate.

A number of studies have been carried out on specific elderly populations in order to determine their nutrition status. Comparisons have been made on nursing-home and free-living elderly in the same location. For example, a study was made in New Jersey of the blood vitamin levels of elderly people living at home or in nursing homes as compared with the levels found in a younger control population (Baker et al, 1979). In general, among the free-living elderly the blood levels of vitamin A and E, and of riboflavin, biotin and pantothenate were adequate, whereas the levels of vitamin C, thiamin, folate and vitamin B_{12} were frequently low (Table 11.1). On the other hand, a different spectrum was found among the institutionalised elderly, who showed low levels of niacin and vitamin B_6 in one-third of the subjects, with less frequent deficiencies of vitamin B_{12}, folate, thiamin and ascorbate. In a similar comparison in Belfast, Northern Ireland (Vir & Love, 1979), nutrient intakes were also examined. The least abundant dietary constituents were potassium, magnesium, vitamin B_6 and vitamin D, and there was mild deficiency of iron, ascorbic acid, thiamin, riboflavin, vitamin B_6 and vitamin D. Comparison between free-living and institutionalised subjects again showed different frequencies of deficiency (Table 12.1). This emphasises the greater risk of certain groups of elderly to nutrient inadequacy.

Are these deficiencies in intake and in blood levels accompanied by any functional deficits? Exton-Smith (1980a) concludes that vitamin deficiencies (based on intakes and blood levels) are commoner in old people than in young people, and he reports evidence that encephalopathies, confusional states and dementia in the elderly are sometimes associated with water-soluble vitamin deficiencies, especially in association with infections and other stresses. This suggests that the marginal nutritional status of many elderly people can become acutely deficient under conditions of stress.

Regarding causes of malnutrition in the elderly, Exton-Smith (1980b) divides these into primary and secondary. The primary causes include:

Table 11.1 Subnormal blood values obtained in two surveys of the elderly

| Population | Percentage of population with subnormal values | | | | | | | |
| | Vitamin C | | Folate | | Thiamin | | B_6 | |
	(1)	(2)	(1)	(2)	(1)	(2)	(1)	(2)
Free-living	24	23	9	48	25	13	18	43
Nursing-home	4	56	20	28	4	11	37	63
Hospitalised	—	41	—	37	—	11	—	29

(1) Data of Baker et al (1979) on 146 free-living and 327 nursing-home elderly in New Jersey
(2) Data of Vir & Love (1979) on 53 free-living, 26 nursing home and 97 hospitalised elderly in Belfast, Northern Ireland

1. Ignorance of the need for a balanced diet
2. Restriction of the range of available foods because of poverty
3. Social isolation, reducing the interest in eating, as seen in a higher frequency of anaemia and of low leukocyte ascorbic acid levels in men living alone, which can be reversed by congregate feeding
4. Physical disability, restricting the capacity to purchase varied foods, and resulting in a lower intake of nutrients by housebound elderly as compared with active elderly.

Malnutrition can also be secondary to malabsorption, which affects especially the fat-soluble vitamins, folic acid and vitamin B_{12}. Alcoholism can cause malnutrition through replacing foodstuffs as an energy source and also by reducing absorption of nutrients, especially folic acid. Finally, older people are often treated chronically with therapeutic drugs, some of which interfere with nutrient utilisation. Thus anticonvulsant drugs can lead to vitamin D deficiency.

INTERVENTIONS IN FEEDING OF THE ELDERLY

Target populations

From long experience of the nutritional status of the elderly in England, Exton-Smith (1980b) has identified groups of elderly at special risk of malnutrition. These include socially isolated individuals, those with a physical disability contributing to isolation, very old men living alone, and those with depression and other mental disorders. He points out that housebound people represent 8 per cent of those over 65 years of age in England, which thus amounts of 650 000 people in a national population of all ages of 50 million. The majority of cases of malnutrition will be found in the housebound groups, and interventions here will be the most effective.

Experience with interventions

Once a target group (e.g. the housebound) has been identified, the quality of a person's diet can be assessed roughly by recording the major food classes consumed (Marr et al, 1961). The nature of the intervention will depend on the circumstances. Meals on wheels can be used for those confined to their houses, while congregate feeding is more appropriate for those who are more mobile, since it has a socialising effect. In order to have a significant impact on the nutrition of the elderly person, Exton-Smith (1980b) reckons four meals a week should be provided. The practice of providing supplements (e.g. vitamins in pill form) has not yet been sanctioned by clinical trial.

The American experience has been less targeted to specific vulnerable groups among the elderly. Food as meals was provided by Congress in 1972 through an amendment (Title VII) to the Older Americans Act of 1965. At first, the programme provided congregate feeding. Subsequent amendments of this act led to both home-delivered and congregate meals, and currently nearly two million American elderly are enrolled in these programmes (Opinion Research Corporation and Kirschner Associates, 1983). Posner (1979) has analysed the impact of this programme on the elderly in the Boston area. She discusses the ideal planning process, starting with identifying the nature of the problem, then looking at the various alternative solutions, proceeding to implementation of the most promising solution and finally evaluation of the programme, this last being regarded as an integral and important component in the planning process, not an afterthought. She emphasises that optimally the impact of a programme should be first evaluated for nutritional status of the population under study, the intake of nutrients likely to be obtained from the intervention and the effect of the programme on the nutrition awareness of the participants before and after the intervention.

In spite of shortcomings, the nutrition program in the Boston area received commendation from its recipients, but this was more because of social interaction resulting from congregate feeding than from nutritional benefits that might accrue from the few meals eaten or because of an impact of the programme on food-purchasing habits of the recipients. A small but significant point is that special ethnic or therapeutic dietary needs of potential participants were not met by this programme. The author emphasises the need for much more research into behavioural and social factors associated with nutritional services for the ageing, and into human services and their delivery to the elderly. Better profiles of different types of elderly who participate in such programmes are required. For these various objectives new methodologies and criteria need to be developed in future evaluations.

It was unfortunate that this Boston survey of the impact of Title VII in the Boston area did not include an assessment of changes in nutritional status, physical performance and health as a result of the dietary intervention. This has, in fact, been performed on a limited group of recipients of the Title VII congregate meal program in Missouri (Kohrs, 1976). Nutritional status and health evaluated by biochemical and clinical examination appear to have been better in the recipients than among non-participating elderly. However, Posner (1979) criticises this study because of lack of evidence of comparability of the participant and non-participant groups.

Other surveys of nutritional impact have also been made in the US on a variety of populations (Caliendo & Smith, 1981; Grandjean et al, 1981; Harrill et al, 1981; Kim et al, 1984). These evaluations tend to show that the programme improved intakes of nutrients in general, especially of some. Regarding the comprehensiveness of the programmes, there was evidence of under-representation of low-income elderly poor and the socially isolated. An extensive study of most aspects of the programme has been made by Opinion Research Corporation and Kirschner Associates (1983). This provides many aspects of both congregate and home feeding of the elderly, including the numbers in each category participating, the impact of the nutrition educational component of the programme, the effect of the programme on health, both perceived and real, the nutritional quality and acceptability of the meals, their sanitary status and the preservation of food quality during preparation and transportation.

The USA also provides a Food Stamp Program for the non-institutionalised elderly, and this has been evaluated in the National Food Consumption Surveys which show that participation in this programme is extensive and increasing. Blanchard et al (1982) made a study of the impact on the nutrition of the recipients of food stamps and concluded that nutrient intake was in general improved, significantly so in the case of calcium. Importantly, following the provision of cash instead of food stamps, the recipients responded by increasing their intakes of calcium, protein, ascorbic acid and thiamin.

Future intervention programmes should identify nutritionally vulnerable target groups within the elderly population. Such interventions must be monitored for efficacy from the start of the programme and cost-effectiveness demonstrated by improved health and function as well as better nutrient intakes and biochemical indices of nutrient adequacy. This will especially involve devising methods of improving the nutrient status of housebound old people living alone, usually the least accessible group. Nutritional services to these should be part of a drive for improved social circumstances, although the provision of adequate numbers of meals to add significantly to the nutrient intake of this group may prove to be very difficult. A second subset of elderly who could be monitored for nutritional status are those in nursing homes. This captive population can be better surveyed, and it would indeed be desirable to evaluate the benefits of good nutritional status to health and function (see Table 11.1).

SUMMARY

Ageing is a phenomenon of the whole of adult life, with progressive loss of tissue function and eventual accumulation of degenerative diseases. The role of nutrition in moderating these processes involves more than determining the levels of essential nutrients to be consumed, but also requires decisions about desirable levels of other non-essential food consitituents, including dietary fibre, and the role of interactions between various nutrients. We are only at the beginning of understanding how long-term nutritional habits, in combination with other lifestyle factors such as regular exercise, may conspire to minimise age-related loss of tissue function and to limit the development of chronic ailments. Nevertheless, evidence from animal studies and from the role of nutritional factors in one major age-related degenerative condition, namely osetoporosis, shows that nutrition has a part to play.

The second aspect of nutrition and ageing is the practical problem of providing adequate levels of nutrients for those who are already old. Here, also, the objective should be to preserve function, but there is little solid evidence on which to base allowances for nutrients in successive decades of later life. Since intakes of many nutrients decline with the diminishing appetite of increasing age, we must ask whether a significant number of the elderly consume less than their needs of essential nutrients. In this context we should recognise the emergence with progressive ageing of target groups who are especially vulnerable to submaintenance intakes of nutrients. Whereas many elderly people remain fit and active into their eighties, those who live alone, are disabled, or have a degree of mental confusion provide the housebound population whose nutrient intake is especially low. They are also least accessible for distribution of supplementary meals which must be made available several times a week and be consumed in order to make a significant contribution to the nutrient intake of this group.

In order to rectify some of these difficulties, more attention has to be paid to nutrition evaluation of subsets of elderly population. Such evaluations will require the provision by further research of standards of nutritional normality applicable specifically to older people, and the identification of the relationship of nutritional status to bodily functions, perhaps with the development of a composite index of functional ageing comparable to the indices of growth and development for the child. Conclusions about desirable nutritional habits among the elderly should also be made in the context of other lifestyle factors such as exercise and the mental stimulation provided by the environment, both of which can be positive factors for nutrient intake.

REFERENCES

Aloia J F, Cohn A H, Babu, T, Abesamis C, Kalici N, Ellis K 1978a Skeletal mass and body composition in marathon runners. Metabolism 27: 1793–1796

Aloia J F, Cohn S H, Ostuni J A, Crane R, Ellis K 1978b Prevention of involutional bone loss by exercise. Annals of Internal Medicine 89: 356–358

American Society for Clinical Nutrition 1979 Report of the task force on the evidence relating six dietary factors to the nation's health. American Journal of Clinical Nutrition 32: 2621–2748

American Society for Clinical Nutrition 1982 Evidence relating selected vitamins and minerals to health and disease in the elderly population of the United States. American Journal of Clinical Nutrition 36: 977–1086

Anand C R, Linkswiler H M 1976 Effect of protein intake on calcium balance of young men given 500 mg calcium daily. Journal of Nutrition 104: 695–700

Andrews J, Letcher M, Brook M 1969 Vitamin C supplementation in the elderly: 17-month trial in an old persons' home. British Medical Journal ii: 416–418

Baker H, Frank O, Thind I S, Jaslow J P, Louria D B 1979 Vitamin profiles in elderly persons living at home or in nursing homes versus profiles in healthy young subjects. Journal of the American Geriatrics Society 27: 444–4501

Blanchard L, Butler J S, Doule P et al 1982 Food stamp SSI/elderly cashout demonstration evaluation. Final Report. Food and Nutrition Service. United States Department of Agriculture

Burr M L, Hurley R J, Sweetman P M 1975 Vitamin C supplementation of old people with low blood levels. Gerontologia Clinica 17: 236–243

Caliendo M A, Smith J 1981 Preliminary observations on the dietary status of participants in the Title III-C meal program. Journal of Nutrition for the Elderly 3: 21–39

Callard R E 1977 Changes in mouse lymphocyte activity with age. Interdisciplinary Topics in Gerontology 11:63–69, Karger, Basel

Cheng A H R, Gomez A, Gergan J G, Lee T C, Monckeberg F, Chichester C O 1978 Comparative nitrogen balance study between young and aged adults using three levels of protein intake from a combination of wheat-soy-milk-mixture. American Journal of Clinical Nutrition 31: 12–22

Cohn S H, Vartsky D, Yasumura S, Sawitsky A, Zanze I, Vaswani A, Ellis K J 1980 Compartmental body composition based on total body nitrogen, potassium, and calcium. American Journal of Physiology 239: E524–530

Debry G, Bleyer R, Martin J M 1977 Nutrition of the elderly. Journal of Human Nutrition 31: 195–204

Department of Health and Social Security: A nutrition survey of the elderly 1979 Reports Health Society Subj. No. 16. HMSO, London

Dibble M V, Brin M, Thiele V F, Peel A, Chen N, McMullen E 1967 Evaluation of the nutritional status of elderly subjects with a comparison between fall and spring. Journal of the American Geriatrics Society 15: 1031–1061

Diet, Nutrition and Cancer Committee 1982 Diet, nutrition and cancer report. National Research Council, Washington D C

Everitt A V 1971 Food intake, growth and the aging of collagen in rat tail tendon. Gerontologia 17: 98–104

Everitt A V, Seedsman G C, Barrows C H 1980 The effect of hypophysectomy and continuous food restriction, begun at ages 70 and 400 days, on collagen, aging, proteinuria, incidence of pathology and longevity in the male rat. Mech. Age Development 12: 161–172

Exton-Smith A N 1977 Proceedings of the Royal Society of Medicine 70: 615–621

Exton-Smith A N 1980a Vitamins. In: Exton-Smith A N, Caird F I (eds) Metabolic and nutritional disorders in the elderly. Wright, Bristol, p 26–38

Exton-Smith A N 1980b Nutritional status: diagnosis and prevention of malnutrition. In: Exton-Smith A N, Caird F I (eds) Metabolic and nutritional disorders in the elderly. Wright, Bristol, p 66–76

Exton-Smith A N, Caird F I (eds) 1980. Metabolic and nutritional disorders in the elderly. John Wright, Bristol

Exton-Smith A N, Stanton B R 1965 Report of an investigation into the diets of elderly women living alone. King Edward's Hospital Fund, London

Forbes G B, Reina J C 1970 Adult lean body mass declines with age: some longitudinal observations. Metabolism 19: 653–663

Garn S M 1978 Bone loss and aging. In: Farmer F A (ed) Nutrition and the aged. University of Calgary Press, Alberta, p 73–90

Gersovitz M, Motil K, Munro H N, Scrimshaw N S, Young V R 1982 Human protein requirements: assessment of the adequacy of the current recommended dietary allowance for dietary protein in elderly men and women. American Journal of Clinical Nutrition 35: 6–14

Gersovitz M, Munro H N, Udall J, Young V R 1980 Albumin synthesis in young and elderly subjects using a new stable isotope methodology: response to level of protein intake. Metabolism 29: 1075–1086

Grandjean A C, North L L, Kara G G, Smith J L, Schaefer A E 1981 Nutritional status of elderly participants in a congregate meal program. Journal of the American Dietetic Association 78: 324–329

Gregerman R I 1967 The age related alteration of thyroid function and thyroid hormone metabolism in man. In: Gitman (ed) Endocrines and aging. Thomas, Springfield, IL, ch 13

Guigoz Y, Munro H N 1985 Health maintenance and longevity: nutrition. In: Finch C E, Schneider E L (eds) Handbook of the biology of aging, 2nd edn, Van Nostrand-Reinhold, New York (in press)

Harrill Il Bowski M, Kylen A, Wemple R R 1981 The nutritional status of congregate meal recipients. Aging 36: 311–312

Heaney R P, Gallagher J C, Johnston C C, Neer R, Parfitt A M, Wheedon G D 1982 Calcium nutrition and bone health in the elderly. American Journal of Clinical Nutrition 36: 986–1013

Heaney R P, Recker R R 1982 Effects of nitrogen, phosphorus and caffeine in calcium balance in women. Journal of Laboratory and Clinical Medicine 99: 46–55

Heaney R P, Recker R R, Saville P D 1978 Menopausal changes in calcium balance performance. Journal of Laboratory and Clinical Medicine 92: 953–963

Horsman A, Gallagher J C, Simpson M, Nordin B E C 1977 Prospective trial of oestrogen and calcium in postmenopausal women. British Medical Journal ii: 789–792

Horsman A, Jones M, Francis R, Nordin C 1983 The effect of estrogen dose on postmenopausal bone loss. New England Journal of Medicine 309: 1405–1407

Kim K, Kohrs M B, Twork R, Grier M R 1984 Dietary calcium intakes of elderly Korean Americans. Journal of the American Dietetic Association 84: 164–169

Kohrs M B 1976 Influences of the congregate meal program in Central Missouri on dietary practices and nutritional status of participants. Jefferson City, MO, Lincoln University, Department of Agriculture and Natural Resources, Human Nutrition Program

Korenchevsky V 1961 Physiological and pathological aging. Hafner, New York

Kritchevsky D 1979 Diet, lipid metabolism and aging. Federation Proceedings 38: 2001–2006

Krolner B, Toft B, Nielsen S P, Tondevold E 1983 Physical exercise as prophylaxis against involutional vertebral bone loss: a controlled trial. Clinical Science 64: 541–546

Matkovic V, Kostial K, Simonovic I, Buzina R, Brodavec A, Nordin B E C 1979 Bone status and fracture rates in two regions of Yugoslavia. American Journal of Clinical Nutrition 32: 540–549

McCay C M, Maynard L A, Sperling G, Barnes L L 1939 Retarded growth, life span, ultimate body size and age changes in the albino rat after feeding diets restricted in calories. Journal of Nutrition 18: 1–13

McGandy R B, Barrows C H, Spanias A, Meredith A, Stone J L, Norris A H 1966 Nutrient intakes and energy expenditure in men of different ages. Journal of Gerontology 21: 581–587

Munro H N 1964a An introduction to nutritional aspects of protein metabolism. In: Munro H N, Allison J B (eds) Mammalian protein metabolism, vol 2. Academic Press, New York, p 3–39

Munro H N 1964b General aspects of the regulation of protein metablism by diet and by hormones. In: Munro H N, Allison J B (eds) Mammalian protein metabolism, vol 1. Academic Press, New York, p 381–481

Munro H N 1981 Nutrition and ageing. British Medical Bulletin 37: 83–88

Munro H N 1984 Nutrition-related problems of middle age. Proceedings of the Nutrition Society (England and Scotland) 43: 281–288

Munro H N, Young V R 1978 Urinary excretion of N^{t}-methyl-histidine (3-methylhistidine): a tool to study metabolic responses in relation to nutrient and hormonal status in health and disease in man. American Journal of Clinical Nutrition 31: 1608–1614

Oliver R F 1981 Diet and coronary heart disease. British Medical Bulletin 37: 49–58

Opinion Research Corporation and Kirschner Associates 1983 An evaluation of the nutrition services for the elderly. Administration for the Aging, Department of Health and Human Services, Washington DC

Parfitt A M, Gallagher J C, Heaney R P, Johnston C C, Neer R, Wheedon G D 1982 Vitamin D and bone health in the elderly. American Journal of Clinical Nutrition 36: 1014–1031

Posner B M 1979 Nutrition and the elderly. Lexington Books, Lexington, MA

Recker R R, Saville P D, Heaney R P 1977 Effect of estrogens and calcium carbonate on bone loss in postmenopausal women. Annals of Internal Medicine 87: 649–655

Recommended Dietary Allowances 1980 9th revised ed. National Academy of Sciences, Washington

Riggs B L, Wahner H W, Seeman E, Offord K P, Dunn W L, Mazess R B, Johnson K A, Melton L J 1982 Changes in bone mineral density of the proximal femur and spine with aging. Differences between the postmenopausal and senile osteoporosis syndromes. Journal of Clinical Investigation 70: 716–723

Shils M E 1980 Nutrition and neoplasia. In: Goodhart R S, Shils M E (eds) Modern nutrition in health and disease, 6th edn. Lea & Febiger, Philadelphia

Shock N W 1972 Energy metabolism, caloric intake and physical activity of the aging. In: Carlson J A (ed) Nutrition in old age. 10th Symposium of the Swedish Nutrition Foundation. Almquist & Wiksell, Uppsala, p 12–23

Silverstone F A, Brandfonbrener M, Shock N W, Yiengst M J 1975 Age differences in the intravenous glucose tolerance tests and the response to insulin. Journal of Clinical Investigation 36: 504–514

Smith E L, Reddan W, Smith P E 1981 Physical activity and calcium modalities for bone mineral increase in aged women. Medicine and Science in Sports and Exercise 13: 60–64

Spencer H, Kramer L, Osis D, Norris C 1978 Effect of a high protein (meat) intake on calcium metabolism in man. American Journal of Clinical Nutrition 31: 2167–2180

Steen G B, Isaksson B, Svanberg A 1979 Body composition at 70 and 75 years of age: a longitudinal population study. Journal of Clinical and Experimental Gerontology 1: 185–200

Stiedemann M, Jansen C, Harrill I 1978 Nutritional status of elderly men and women. Journaal of the American Dietetic Association 73: 132–139

Ten-State Survey: Highlights 1972 DHEW publication No (HSM) 72–8134 US Department of Health, Education and Welfare, Washington DC

Uauy R, Winterer J C, Bilmazes C, Haverberg L W, Scrimshaw N S, Munro H N, Young V R 1978 The changing pattern of whole body protein metabolism in aging humans. Journal of Gerontology 33: 663–675

Vir S C, Love A H G 1979 Nutritional status of institutionalised and non-institutionalized aged in Belfast, Northern Ireland. American Journal of Clinical Nutrition 32: 1934–1947

Weindruch R H, Kristie J A, Chaney K E, Walford R L 1979 Influence of controlled dietary restriction on immunologic function and aging. Federation Proceedings 38: 2007–2016

Zanni E, Calloway D H, Zezulka A Y 1979 Protein requirements of elderly men. Journal of Nutrition 109: 513–524

Prevention of pressure sores

INTRODUCTION

Pressure sores are defined as sores which develop from a prolonged period of ischaemia in the tissue (Barton, 1974) and a number of other terms are used interchangeably to describe them — most commonly bedsores, or decubitus ulcers. Decubitus is a derivation from the Greek to lie down, so that the latter two terms relate to the fact that pressure sores are common in the bedridden. In the international classification of diseases, the pressure sores classification (class 707 0) is headed Decubitus ulcer, and includes the terms pressure ulcer and plaster ulcer. *Pressure* sore or ulcer more accurately reflects the contemporary belief that the ischaemia, necrosis and eventual ulceration of tissue arises as a result of pressure (Daniel et al 1978).

Barton & Barton (1981) divide pressure sores into two classes — those due to pressure alone, and those due to local endothelial cell damage arising from a number of factors. A variety of classifications are described in the literature; Forrest (1980) lists six types of sores ranging from superficial/moist, to deep and cavitating (Fig.12.1), and Cooney & Reuler (1983) list four. Daniel et al (1978) propose a classification of five grades of pressure sores, based on analysis of the literature, which represents a developmental grading presupposing that a sore may progress from grade 1 to grade 5:

Grade 1. A skin area of erythema or induration overlying a bony prominence.

Grade 2. A skin area of superficial ulceration extending into the dermis.

Grade 3. An ulcer extending into the subcutaneous tissue, but not into muscle.

Grade 4. A deep ulcer extending through muscle to the bony prominance.

Grade 5. An extensive ulcer with widespread extension along bursae or into joints or body cavities.

The aetiology of pressure sores is less clear than many assume. Whilst pressure is seen to be the most significant contributing factor, as the term pressure sore implies, it is not the only one, and in some cases not the primary cause.

The prolonged ischaemia which precipitates the development of the sore

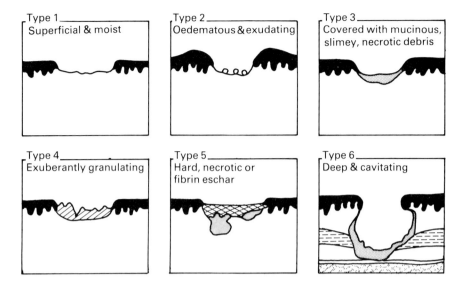

Fig. 12.1 Classification of the types of pressure sores (Forrest, 1980)

most frequently, however, arises as a result of pressure on the tissue which exceeds the capillary pressure of 15–40 mm Hg and thus occludes capillary circulation (Dinsdale, 1974; Kosiak et al, 1958; Agris & Spira, 1979). Reactive hyperaemia develops from the vasodilation caused by an active inflammatory process. If perfusion of the tissues and the removal of toxic by-products takes place fairly rapidly as a result of relieving the pressure, the initial tissue damage may be reversible, but if the pressure is maintained, irreversible damage may follow and necrosis and ulceration can occur in 1–6 hours (Judson, 1983). Agris & Spira (1979) suggest that short periods of intense pressure are equally as damaging as long periods of less pressure. A constant pressure of 70 mm Hg applied for longer than two hours was found by Dinsdale (1974) to produce irreversible damage, but little changes occurred up to pressures of 240 mm Hg if this pressure was regularly relieved. Daniel et al (1978) question the evidence available to substantiate that pressure is the vital causal factor. Citing the work of Kosiak et al (1958), they note that continuous pressures of 100 mm Hg for up to 12 hours, and of 150 mm Hg for 11 hours, did not result in pressure sores. They question they validity of the pressure–ischaemia pathogenesis of pressure sores, and urge for further experimental studies to clarify the various casual factors.

Barton & Barton (1981) suggest that every nurse knows there are circumstances where despite pressure being relieved, and every care taken, severe sores will develop, and other important contributing factors have been identified. Paralysis, sensory loss, reduction in the level of consciousness, circulatory disorders, fever, anaemia, malnutrition, incontinence, mental apathy, heavy sedation and anaesthesia are reported as predisposing factors by Exton-

Smith (1976), and shearing forces and friction have been found to directly cause sores by Reichel (1958). Dinsdale (1974) also concluded from his study that friction played a major part in sore development. Cooney & Reuler (1981) discuss the other major contributing factor — the presence of moisture, notably in incontinence of faeces and/or urine, or excessive perspiration, suggesting that this increases the risk of pressure sore formation fivefold.

Whilst pressure is currently seen to be the single most crucial causative factor, the precise mechanism by which it produces tissue necrosis clinically remains unresolved, and Dinsdale (1973,1974) suggests that it is at present unwise to conclude that the pressure–ischaemia relationship is always the greatest causal factor, noting that the different pressures required to produce skin necrosis do not correlate closely with the pressure exerted on the human skin during normal activites of daily living. The relative contributions of the other factors mentioned — shearing forces, friction, moisture, loss of sensation, nutrition etc. — are still not clear, and further experimental studies are needed before the aetiology of pressure sores can be clearly understood (Daniel et al 1981)

THE INCIDENCE AND PREVALENCE OF PRESSURE SORES

Despite the variance in describing and classifying pressure sores, and in the understanding of their aetiology, there is no dissent from the view that the occurrence of pressure sores, particularly in the elderly, is a problem of major concern throughout the world. They have plagued humankind in all ages — pressure sores were seen on Egyptian mummies by Rowling (1961), and they are referred to in the Bible (Romm et al 1982) on a number of occasions. In 1872, Shaw identified bedsores as a major problem, specifically in young people suffering from the debilitating diseases of the time–tuberculosis, osteomyelitis and chronic renal disease (Shaw, 1872).

Contemporary surveys reveal that the incidence and prevalence of bedsores continues to be a significant problem, and that the majority of sufferers are now elderly, often have changes in mental status, frequently are incontinent, and are unable to be mobile without help (Manley, 1978; Peterson & Bittman, 1971; Walldorf, 1976).

The absolute incidence of pressure sores is difficult to determine, but a number of surveys present similar enough findings on which to generalise. In a questionnaire survey of over ten thousand patients within the Greater Glasgow Health Board Area in Scotland, 8.8 per cent of the patients entered into the study had a lesion which could be identified as a pressure sore, and these were equally prevalent whether patients were nursed at home or in hospital (Barbenel et al 1981). In discussing the findings, Barbenel et al (1977) and Clark et al (1978) estimated that the 8.8 per cent was an underestimate of 2–3 per cent, and later report an even higher prevalence, with a greater proportion of deep sores in a subsequent survey in the Border Health Board Area of Scotland (Barbenel, 1980).

In the Glasgow area, 946 patients (8.8 per cent) had a pressure sore, and 400 of these had at least one severe sore. In both of the surveys, the highest prevalence of pressure sores was in the elderly, and incontinence and immobility increased the risk of developing sores. In Denmark, Peterson & Bittman (1971) found a prevalence of pressure sores of 43.1 per 100 000 population. Fifty-nine percent of patients with sores were hospitalised, and of those in hospital, 63 percent developed the sores whilst in hospital.

Many studies of hospital patients have been carried out, and the incidence of pressure sores for hospitalised patients has been generally found to be between 3 and 8 per cent. Manley (1978) found an incidence of 3 per cent and Peterson & Bittman (1971) of 4.5 per cent in general hospitals. In a study of acute and extended care hospitals in and near Baltimore in the USA, 10 per cent of patients in the extended care hospitals had pressure sores, and 21 per cent of patients admitted to these extended care hospitals from acute areas during the study period had pressure sores on admission (Read 1981). Twenty to thirty percent of patients in a geriatric hospital in England were found to have pressure sores in an unnamed study cited by Barton & Barton (1981) and in the hospital where they work, little sex differences in incidence were apparent in a sample of 500 patients with pressure sores.

In Barton & Barton's (1981) sample, 61 per cent of sores occurred in the sacrococcygeal region, 14 per cent on the heels, and 20 per cent in other sites. Reuler & Cooney (1981) suggest that 96 per cent of pressure sores occur in the lower part of the body, mainly in the sacral and coccygeal area, the ischial tuberosities and over the greater trochanter. Figure 12.2 shows the common areas susceptible to pressure sores. In a study of pressure sores in a Swedish hospital, Ek and Boman (1982) found 71 patients suffering from one or more pressure sores in one week (4% of the hospital population), and a total of 109 sores were observed. As Table 12.1 shows, the majority of sores occurred in

Table 12.1 Site distribution of sores occurring in a Swedish Hospital (Ek & Boman, 1981)

Site	%
Sacrum	35
T. ischiadium	16
Remainder	15
T. calcanei	11
Trochanter major	7
Cristailianca	7
Ear	3
Malleolus	3
Cubitus	2
Shoulder	2
	101

$n = 109$

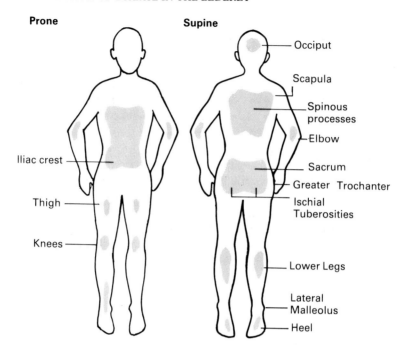

Fig. 12.2 Common sites of pressure sores (Cooney & Reuler, 1983)

the lower part of the body. They also found that more women than men developed sores, and that the majority of patients were over 65, with those in the 80–84 range predominating. Limited mobility and incontinence were significantly associated with pressure sores.

The majority of the surveys reported confirm the subjective suspicious of the experienced nurse:
1. The greatest incidence is in he chronically ill and the elderly
2. The greatest prevalence is in those who have limitation in mobility
3. Most sores occur below the level of the umbilicus.

Epedemiologically, the elderly, the chronically ill and the hospitalised represent the three major groups at risk to pressure sores, and the incidence and prevalence of pressure sores in itself demands that the problem be taken seriously.

THE EFFECTS OF THE PROBLEM

The direct effects of a pressure sore on the individual patient can be approached in two ways: the pathological sequelae, and the effects on the person's quality of daily life. Whilst analysis and limited research into the former by medical practitioners exist, little appears in the literature by them, or by nurses, on the latter.

Medical complications which may arise following onset of a pressure sore are multiple and may be life-threatening. Cooney & Reuler (1983) discuss the common complications of infection, citing evidence from Galpin et al (1976) which suggests tht most infections secondary to pressure sores are polymicrobial, and Laforce et al (1969) who found that pressure sores which extend into deep structures such as the bowel and bladder may lead to tetanus. Contractures of the limbs and disfigurement are also common complications.

Effects on the individual

In terms of the individual, the effects of succumbing to a pressure sore can be summarised as: pain, extended hospital stay, unnecessary restriction on treatment/rehabilitation regimes, and loss of independence. Little appears in the literature on these problems (which indicates that a wealth of brand-new data exist for would-be researchers!), and discussion of them is subjective and unsubstantiated.

Pain

Whilst pressure sores are more likely to develop in patients with lessened sensation, the pain which patients complain of from pressure sores appears to be a common problem. As well as being painful when the sore is cleaned and dressed, the nature of pressure sores in themselves means that the patient is very often unable to lie or sit in the position which he or she normally finds most comfortable.

Extension of hospital stay

Patients admitted to hospital with acute problems amenable to treatment very often need to remain in hospital long after resolution of the initial problem, until the pressure sore is resolved. Norton et al (1975) found that the duration of hospital stay was much longer in those with pressure sores than in those without, in their in-depth study of geriatric patients. As well as patients remaining in hospital until the sore is healed, hospital stay may be lengthened because presence of the sore prevents them from participating as fully as they could in the planned rehabilitation programme, and thus the return to the target independence level is slowed down. (Shand & McClemont, 1979); Lancet, 1981).

Unnecessary restriction on treatment/rehabilitation regimes

As discussed above, hospital stay may be lengthened because the patient is unable to take part in occupational therapy, physiotherapy, or other rehabilitation regime in some cases of pressure sores. For example, Norton et al (1975) found the presence of pressure sores on the heels restricted the patient's ability to carry out physiotherapy. Heel involvement was seen to prevent the wearing of shoes and can therefore delay walking exercises at a crucial time in the patient's rehabilitation. Bardsley et al (1964) found that 30 patients with pressure sores lost a total of 4874 days from their active rehabilitation programmes over an eighteen-month period.

Effects on the nursing staff

Whilst the major effects of pressure sores are to prolong morbidity, delay rehabilitation, cause death, produce pain and extend the hospital stay (Steffel et al 1980), the effects of their occurrence on the morale and subsequent performance of nurses — the front-line carers or "worker bees of the system" (Tiffany, 1979) — cannot be ignored.

Although Kataria & Datta (1982) consider pressure sores to be challenge to nurses, Shand & McClemont (1979) note how they always involve nursing staff in considerably more work, and Forrest (1980) says that this work is unpleasant, time-consuming, unglamorous and difficult. He further suggests that the appearance of a pressure sore connotes failure to the nurse, and care of the sore becomes stigmatised, often being delegated to the junior members of the nursing team. Trivial though this may appear on first sight, it has important implications. In addition to the initial demoralising effect aroused by the appearance of the sore, and the stigma attached to the patient, tradition also dictates that it is a direct result of inneffective and inadequate nursing. Nightingale (1861), who is still nursing's heroine image, herself wrote that if a patient develops a bedsore, it is the fault of the nurse and not the fault of the disease. Witkowski & Parish (1982) suggest that such a sentiment is often shared by medical practitioners, who assume that they have nothing to offer therapeutically, and delegate total care to the nursing team. The stigma attached to the patient may therefore deepen, with the doctor routinely passing the patient and labelling him or her as a nursing problem.

Romm et al (1982) suggest that, whilst nursing intervention is the crucial determinant of the outcome, nurses can be best motivated to be creative in planning care and giving care of the highest quality, by amending Nightingale's statement to read it is the fault of the nurse, the doctor, and the patient. If the occurrence of a pressure sore continues to be a mark of failure in nursing care alone, and it's future resolution a rather dull, low-status nursing task, then virtual rejection of the patient by other health care workers will continue to be one of the effects of having a pressure sore on the individual.

PREVENTING PRESSURE SORES

Apart from the financial burden created when patients develop pressure sores, which is briefly discussed later in this chapter, the dramatic effects on the patient demand that any preventive measures substantiated should be rigorously pursued. The high incidence and prevalence of pressure sores in the elderly at home and in hospital would seem to suggest that health workers are unable, at the moment, to prevent pressure sores. However, although much of the literature on prevention presents the findings of small-scale studies there is enough evidence to suggest that high-risk patients can be identified and that specific interventions can reduce incidence. Norton et al (1975) report a striking reduction in the incidence of pressure sores in a sample of 100 patients who were identified as being highly at risk, when a programme of frequent turning was carried out, and a number of studies confirm that objectively *identifying* high-risk patients, and *increasing nursing and medical intervention* as soon as these patients are identified will prevent the occurrence of pressure sores in many (Anderson et al, 1982; Stewart & Wharton, 1976).

Whilst there is still an obvious need for further experimental studies which test the effects of nursing and medical preventive strategies and produce prescriptive data, strategies already found to be effective apparently are not being applied in practice. Widespread ignorance of assessment routines to identify those at risk, such as the Norton scale (Norton et al, 1975), exists in the United Kingdom, says Barbenel (1980). He suggests that the arduous and time-consuming turning of patients by hospital and community nurses is impractical if not concentrated on those identified at risk. Systematically identifying high-risk patients thus helps in deploying the limited nursing resources available in the most effective way.

Many nurses practice from a traditional wisdom knowledge base and reject research-based strategies, often seeing them as undermining their own professional integrity. It is therefore not unusual for ward sisters and district nurses to assert that they themselves just know which patients are at risk, and to apply an array of topical applications to skin to prevent pressure sores. Some strategies employed by experienced nurses may well be effective, but need to be substantiated scientifically.

The fact that the incidence of pressure sores is high is therefore probably not indicative that pressure sores are not preventable, but that those measures currently known to prevent them are not being applied.

Primary prevention

The risk of onset of pressure sores can be reduced by identifying high-risk patients, by implementing appropriate nursing and medical interventions and by involving the patient and relevant others in, and teaching them about, these interventions.

Identifying those who are at risk

The best-known, and most often used, scoring system for identifying patients who are at risk is that developed by Norton et al (1975), first published in

Table 12.2 The Norton scoring system to identify patients at risk. (Norton et al, 1975)

PHYS. COND.		MENTAL COND.		ACTIVITY		MOBILITY		INCONTINENT		
Good	4	Alert	4	Ambulant	4	Full	4	Not	4	Total
Fair	3	Apathetic	3	Walk/help	3	Sl. limited	3	Occasional	3	Score
Poor	2	Confused	2	Chairbound	2	V. limited	2	Usually/Ur.	2	
V. Bad	1	Stupor	1	Bed	1	Immobile	1	Doubly	1	

NAME DATE
_____

_____
_____
_____
_____

1962 (Table 12.2). It has been found to be an applicable and sensitive tool by Cooney & Reuler (1983), and has been incorporated in to many nursing assessment formats in the Western world. As Table 12.2. shows, the five basic elements of the Norton scale are:
1. Physical condition
2. Mental condition
3. Activity
4. Mobility
5. Incontinence

Each of these is assessed and given a score from 1 to 4. The patient who is physically and mentally in an extremely poor state would score 1 in each of the five categories, giving a total score of 5 and indicating a serious risk of developing a pressure sore. The fit, active patient could achieve a score of up to 20.

In the study carried out by Norton and her colleagues (which represented a major milestone both in the beginning of research by nurses and in the start of serious enquiry into care of the elderly), a linear relationship between the score of a patient and the incidence of sores became apparent, with the development of a pressure sore being associated with a lower score. A score of 14 or less is said to indicate that the patient is at risk, and patients scoring 12 or less are regarded as being highly at risk and merit extra nursing.

Although adoption of this tool has not become widespread, a large number of nurses now use it, and its predictive value has been tested by nurses and doctors. Goldstone & Roberts (1980), Goldstone & Goldstone (1982) and Anderson et al (1982) all found the Norton score to be an effective predictor. The crucial elements were found to be the physical and incontinence score, and some studies suggest that:

1. Not all of the five elements are needed to predict the possibility of pressure sores developing (Goldstone & Roberts, 1980)

2. Grading the five elements requires more time and knowledge than is generally available (Anderson et al 1982)
3. Rating scales are not generally acceptable to clinical nurses (Crawford, 1979).

Other studies investigating risk factors seem to support Norton et al's system, in that the five factors repeatedly appear to be associated with the eventual occurrence of a sore (e.g. Coswell, 1973; Ek & Boman, 1982).

The use of a tool such as Norton et al's is an important first step in primary prevention, although further research to enhance its predictive value is needed. Goldstone & Goldstone (1982) conclude that the Norton score is a reliable guide in identifying those at risk, even though they found that it tends to overpredict sores where they do not in fact materialise. Barton & Barton (1981) suggest the use of Thermography as a means of identifying those at risk. Despite the usefulness of this, however, it is difficult to use with many elderly patients, and is not yet as practicable as using scoring systems.

Preventive nursing interventions

Apart from Norton et al's work, little valid and reliable evaluation of nursing actions to prevent pressure sores is available. Norton et al found that regular position change was the only action which effectively reduced the incidence of pressure lesions. A number of topical applications were tested, and zinc cream with tincture of benzoin added had some effect when applied to pressure areas, but was not sufficiently significant to be prescriptive. Small clinical trials by other writers suggest various other strategies, but all need further evaluation.

Until further studies are conducted, preventive nursing measures can only be based on a number of principles, and the findings of limited studies. All of these should be equally applicable to hospital patients, and those in their own homes, although the latter group tend to have less access to equipment and pressure-relieving devices, and have to depend on family members or friends to act as carers.

Position change. The rigorous two-hourly turning routines carried out in neurosurgical and paraplegic units have dramatically reduced the incidence and prevalence of pressure sores in these specialties, and Norton et al (1975) found the same when this was used in geriatric wards. The use of a position change chart (Table 12.3) has been found to be useful in many areas. The relief in continuous pressure which this brings makes this the most effective preventive measure which nurses can provide. Whilst the Lancet (1981) and Reed (1981) advocate either the introduction of special turning orderlies, or special nursing teams, it is likely that such approaches lead to fragmentation of care. The elderly need continuity and the opportunity to develop relationships between carers in hospital, and hiving off discreet tasks to various specialist task-performers cannot be seen as desirable. In home care, if family

Table 12.3 Patient Position Change Chart (Norton et al, 1975)

Times	Position
10 a.m./p.m.	Left Side
12 m.d.*/m.n.	Supine
2 p.m./a.m.	Righ Side
4 p.m./a.m.	Left Side
6 p.m.*/a.m.*	Supine
8 p.m./a.m.	Right Side

*It will be noted that using this particular rota the patient is in a convenient position for at least two meals and for washing in the morning.

members or friends are willing, they can be taught by nursing sisters to institute turning regimes.

Beds and bedding. A large majority of those at risk are bedfast, or spend a good deal of time in bed. The mattress and bedding used have been found to be important in prevention. Interior-spring mattresses on sprung beds have been found to produce high interface pressures, and foam mattresses with solid-base beds produce the lowest pressures (Barbenel et al 1981; Barbenel, 1980). For the elderly, 13 cm — thick, low-density foam mattresses on Kings Fund beds are the most suitable, and their relatively short life dictates that a regular assessment and replacement programme should be in operation. Although mattresses at use in the patient's own home are likely to be in better condition than those in hospitals, the provision of bed boards and foam mattresses for high-risk patients nursed at home will reduce the risks. Stiff, rigid waterproof covers in common use have also been found to contribute to the development of sores, and Ferguson-Pell et al (1979) found that a polyurethane-coated knitted cover reduced interface forces.

Coarsely woven drawsheets, with rubber draw macs are condemned by Norton et al (1975), and heavy blankets were found to increase the pressure exerted on pressure areas. The same conclusions can be drawn for wheelchair or chair cushions and covers for those who are chairbound.

Pressure-relieving equipment. A vast array of simple and complex aids to relieving pressure have been developed, and each aid seems to have a group of supporters who assert its virtues and volubly witness to its effectiveness in prevention. Little reliable evidence is available on which aids are most effective for which group of patients with similar characteristics. The general view seems to be that manual position change carried out carefully and regularly by carers is the basic most effective nursing intervention, and that aids may serve to supplement this, and perhaps make it easier, but can never replace it. A brief review of these aids may be useful, but there is an urgent need for clinical research to test comparative effectiveness. A large proportion of the nursing budget in hospital and community services is expended on these devices, yet none of them supplants the constant vigilance needed by the patient and the carers, and careful changing of weight-bearing surfaces.

Many practitioners advocate the use of ripple mattresses of alternating-pressure mattresses, and some small trials suggest that these are effective (Reswick et al, 1976; Steffel et al, 1980), but more data are needed before this conclusion can be accepted as valid. Many designs are now available on the market, all being based on the system of air cells which inflate and deflate alternately underneath the patient in such a way as to relieve pressure on all the body parts under pressure in the course of about ten minutes. They are cheap and easy to use, in both hospital and at home, but studies in the UK repeatedly report poor maintenance, with many mattresses not working properly (Barton & Barton, 1981; Bliss, 1979).

Water beds and mattresses have many supporters, but there is little objective evaluative data which reliably demonstrates their comparative effectiveness. They usually consist of one or more chambers of water covered with thin material on the water surface. The patient lies on this material, and the water displacement causes a state of weightlessness, and thus a reduction in the pressure (Lilla et al 1975.) They are often bulky and difficult to install, particularly at home, require regular servicing and care and are comparatively expensive. The Stryker frame, Foster frame, electric circular bed and tilt table are all examples of beds which can be used to change the patient's position mechanically. They have been generally found to be effective, in that they simply provide the means through which the nurse can move patients with less physical exertion. The Net suspension system is said to distribute body weight equally. All of them are comparatively expensive and bulky. They are, therefore, less useful to patients at home and, because they are different to a conventional bed, are sometimes unnacceptable to patients (Romm et al 1982; Norton et al 1975).

Numerous pads and small aids are also available, many having undergone small controlled clinical trials, but, again, little prescriptive data exists. Use of small aids seems to be determined by the individual preferences of nurses, and further evaluation of these aids is a top priority in nursing research, yet little appears to be in progress. Foam pads and rings are used to relieve pressure on specific points and to provide bridging — that is, to suspend a specific body area between two points. Flotation pads which contain a gel similar in consistency to body fat are used, particularly in chairs, and are said to be comfortable as well as being effective in distributing pressure. Sheepskins and lamb fleeces are used extensively because of their resilience and capacity to absorb moisture which minimises friction and disperses pressure (Reuler & Cooney, 1981).

Whilst mechanical turning beds certainly reduce the shear manual energy required by nurses and carers, and the other aids may well be useful to prevention, it remains to be seen if they are any more effective than providing enough skilled nurses to change the patient's position every two hours and to establish which aids are of the most use for specific patient groups.

Skin care. For many years nurses have used a host of agents on the skin over pressure points for example soap and water rubs, spirit, eau de Cologne and talcum powder but Norton et al (1975) found no justification for vigorous massage or using topical applications, except when incontinence was present, and the majority of study authors on the subject concur with this. Keeping the skin dry, clean, and regularly observing it for any changes in colour or texture is an important preventive activity. When incontinence is present, barrier creams have been found to be useful, and the use of absorbent drawsheets, such as the Kylie sheet, which absorb urine so that the skin is not bathed in it for long periods, have reduced the incidence of pressure sores in small clinical trials. The effectiveness of other topical applications has yet to be demonstrated.

Involving the patient and his or her family in prevention. If the patient is able to become a partner with the carer, prevention can become a more realistic possibility. In hospital, active teaching and involvement of the patient in formulating a written care plan with clearly stated goals can ensure continuity of the plan. If capable, the patient can be taught to carry out regular position changes and, if this is physically impossible, can direct nurses and carers in the execution of the care plan. Similarly, relatives and friends can be taught how to carry out preventive activities and then encouraged to do so in the hospital. Not only does this release nursing time for patients at risk who do not have relatives, but it also may serve to meet emotional and social needs of the patient and relatives alike and is an important pre-discharge strategy which will enable the family to continue care when the patient returns home (Norton et al, 1975).

Methodical care planning. Both in hospital, and in the home, nursing is essentially delivered by a team of nurses rather than a single nurse. It is therefore impractical to assume that a preventive strategy will be maintained, if a plan, and the rationale behind it, is not written down. Norton and her colleagues report that there was an almost total absence of written basic plans for patients in hospital, and that, accordingly, plans were not carried out continuously. Since this 1962 study, individual plans for patients are being increasingly written, and there is now a trend towards sharing these with patients and their relatives, both in hospital and at home. Plans clearly stating the intervention in specific terms and the goals of the intervention can be left with the patient in his home, or at the hospital bedside.

On the basis of current knowledge, the most effective nursing care to prevent pressure sores can be summarised as the reduction of pressure and friction by

1. Changing the position of the patient every two hours
2. Skilful lifting and movement
3. The use of a foam mattress on a firm bed base
4. The use of polyurethane mattress covers
5. Maintaining smooth, wrinkle-free sheets
6. Using lightweight blankets
7. Accurately documenting individual plans of care
8. Sharing these plans with the patient and his or her relatives, and involving them in care

Pressure-relieving devices and mechanical position-changing beds may also be of use, but further research to test their relative effectivenesses is warranted.

Preventive medical interventions

Whilst pressure appears to be the most significant contributory factor, and nursing intervention is largely aimed at resolving this, medical assessment and subsequent action can also reduce the risk of pressure sores developing.

The maintainence of an adequate capillary circulation is fundamental to prevention. Barton & Barton (1981) suggest that the cardiovascular status be assessed, although the majority of elderly patients at risk do not suffer from anaemia or low blood flow states and thus little can be done for them to improve general circulation, ACTH appears to protect the integrity of the capillary vascular epithelium (Barton, 1977).

A poor nutritional state may predispose to the development of pressure sores, particularly protein and iron deficiencies. Assessment of nutritional status and measures to resolve deficiencies are therefore of use.

The patient himself or herself is a vital resource in prevention, but is often unable to participate in the preventive plan because he or she is either unaware of it, or does not understand the reasons behind it. Purposeful and active information-giving to those patients who are able to be involved is in itself an effective medical intervention. It also frequently serves to give credibility to the teaching initiatives of nurses (Ley et al, 1980).

Primary prevention of pressure sores has traditionally been the task of nursing, and generating knowledge about the effects of pressure and evaluating the outcomes of the various nursing interventions aimed at relieving this pressure is an appropriate task for nurses. However, pressure alone has not been found to be the sole cause of pressure sores, and shared work on prevention between doctors, nurses and paramedical workers is needed.

Secondary and tertiary prevention are, of course, difficult to achieve, and much unnecessary suffering, cost and work can be avoided if the problem of prevention of onset is pursued vigorously and systematically.

Secondary prevention

In discussing secondary prevention related to pressure sores, the WHO definition mentioned in chapter 1 is more appropriate than the terms of screening and case-finding. Pressure sores are usually recognised by a health worker if they exist, and the majority of patients with pressure lesions are likely to be receiving health care in one form or another, and thus case-finding does not appear to be a priority. Similarly, an overlap exists between secondary prevention and tertiary prevention, in that the reduction of the prevalence of pressure sores depends upon effective clinical intervention.

Shortening the course and duration of pressure sores in an individual demands effective treatment, and it is difficult to identify an area other than that of the treatment of pressure sores in which more confusion exists. Between 70 and 90 per cent of sores are superficial and are said to be amenable to non-surgical intervention (Reuler & Cooney, 1981). A vast array of treatment regimes exist for the treatment of superficial pressure sores, (i.e. in addition to surgical procedures for grade 4 and 5 sores) and there is a wealth of advice on treatment. Little is available, however, that is based on objective evidence.

The principles of treatment stem from those of prevention and relief of pressure, and keeping the area clean and dry–plus specific treatment of the sore and systemic assessment and treatment. Specific topical approaches are extensive, but little objective evidence of their effectiveness exists. Fernie & Dornan (1976) are critical of the large number of short-term, small-sampled, clinical trials into topical treatment of pressure sores, and describe how numerous claims for new and effective methods of treatment have arisen from inadequate trials, and how specific regimes all quickly accrue enthusiastic advocates. The literature reveals many reports on limited clinical trials of topical applications often devoid of significant controls.

Topical treatment of a pressure sore can be based on the principles applied to wound-healing generally, and should be determined by the extent and depth of the sore.

Initial skin changes

Erythema can be resolved by relieving pressure, and topical applications are superfluous. Early detection of erythema and immediate action can prevent any further damage. Superficial blistering again can be reversed if action is taken early, but a risk of infection arises, and keeping the area clean may lessen the risk.

Superficial skin breakdown

Relief from pressure, débridement of necrotic tissue and the suppression of infection are the only interventions currently found to be effective in promoting healing of pressure sores, and the goal of providing the most suitable conditions for the healing process is at present the best that can be done. The majority of pressure sores in the elderly fall into this superficial category.

Deep pressure sores

Topical applications are of no use when a sore reaches this stage, the prevention of infection becoming the major goal until surgical action can be taken. Occlusive dressings to reduce the risk of infection, applied using an aseptic technique, are the usual approach until plastic surgery is possible.

Other topical applications and approaches are at present unproven, and cannot be validly advocated until this situation is changed.

Systematic treatment can be based on thorough medical assessment and treatment of any relevant disorders. Particular attention to nutritional status and the possibility of infection is necessary. Protein, iron and ascorbic acid deficiency appears to retard healing, and some limited studies report a speeding-up of the healing process if these deficiencies are reversed (Mulholland, 1943; Taylor et al 1974). Cohen (1978) found that zinc sulphate reduced healing time. An inadequate dietary intake in the elderly patient often compounds the problem, and it is sometimes neccessary to feed him or her via a naso-gastric tube, or parently, if resolution of the sore will allow the patient either to return to a satisfactory quality of life or to become involved in rehabilitative activities which will eventually lead to this. Local infection may require antibiotics, and systemic infection, although not common, is a risk and is often the cause of mortality.

Reducing the prevalence of pressure sores is likely to remain a problem until clinical research on the effectiveness of treatment develops, as all too often treatment is based on the subjective preference and gut feelings of practitioners. There are variations in approaches between individual nurses in a single team, and between doctors. Forrest (1980) describes a standard treatment programme for pressure sores incorporating available knowledge, which could act as a useful guide to practitioners (Table 12.4) and adequately summarises this discussion.

THE COSTS OF PREVENTION

The costs of pressure sores

The occurrence of a pressure sore creates a need for extra resources and increases the length of stay in hospital, or the continuation of community care at home. The absolute costs are difficult to determine, but a number of estimates have been made. In the United Kingdom, it has been said that the annual cost to the health service is £60–100 million, and this is regarded by some to be a very conservative estimate. Eldberg et al (1973) suggest that the treatment of each patient with a pressure sore in the United States costs $15–30 000 depending on the type of sore, and Vistres (1979) sets the cost at about $14 000 per patient. Similar sums are estimated in Scandanavian countries.

The human costs are less amenable to quantification, yet represent the centre of the problem. Apart from significant morbidity and mortality and the symptomatic manifestations of pressure sores, their occurrence often presents new, major problems to elderly people and their families, who were already facing difficulties in maintaining a daily life pattern. In the community, the demands on the caring relative are vastly increased and the older person's feeling of dependency and decline become heightened.

In both human and economic terms, the costs of pressure sores warrant as much preventive effort as the more fashionable health problems such as smoking, for example.

Table 12.4 Pressure sore treatment guide (Forrest, 1980)

AIM OF TREATMENT
To obtain healing of the ulcer or to prepare it for grafting (or closure) by treating inflammation or infection, removing contamination and improving tissue nutrition and local immune defences as well as protecting the wound surface from trauma or re-infection.

GENERAL PRINCIPLES OF TREATMENT
Treatment of pressure sores is difficult and depressing. Skill and experience is required. General nursing care and prevention are the best measures. Improved nutrition annd treatment of sepsis or metabolic disease forms the basis for specific wound treatment.
Topical agents do not heal wounds. They may treat local infections, remove contamination or protect the ulcer surface. All too often they cause allergy and should be used carefully and for as short a period of time as possible. There are many such agents available and this programme should be used as a guide to selection and use of suitable substances.

METHODS
a. Improvement of the patient's general condition:
 1. Improve nutrition, increase protein and energy intake;
 2. Treat anaemia;
 3. Treat vitamin and trace element deficiency (zinc, vitamin C, etc.);
 4. Correct metabolic abnormalities: diabetes mellitus, thyrotoxicosis, if possible reduce dosage of corticosteroids;
 5. Improve circulation and tissue nutrition: vasodilator drugs may be tried. Haemodilution may be useful in pre-gangrene.
 6. Additional treatment: diuretics to control oedema, treatment of heart failure, reduction of dose of immuno-suppressive or cytotoxic drugs, etc.

METHODS (continued)
b. Classification of the ulcer:
 Six types of wound are recognised:
c. Local treatment of the ulcer:
 1. Treatment of inflammation: Local inflammation delays healing. Remove contamination, foreign body and infection. In some cases surgical debridement;
 2. Treatment of infection: systemic antibiotics where indicated. In superficial infection: dextranomer;
 3. Remove necrotic tissue or debris: Surgical debridement. Short trial of enzyme agent followed by wet compresses or (if the ulcer is exudating) dextranomer;
d. Ulcer treatment:
 Type 1: Keep moist & pliable with saline compresses.
 Type 2: Exudation allows secondary infection. Inflamed & oedematous. Remove oedema & inflammation with dextranomer which promotes granulation.
 Type 3: The film of slimy debris is difficult to remove manually.
 Enzymes may have to be used. When the surface is clean use wet compresses or (in exudating wounds) dextranomer;
 Type 4: Surgical removal of lumps of granulation, cauterisation with silver nitrate;
 Type 5: Surgical debridement followed either by a short treatment with enzymes or saline compresses (if the wound is clean);
 Type 6: Surgical debridement. Thereafter enzymes or dextranomer if required. The latter stimulates granulation and prepares the ulcer for grafting or a rotation flap.
 Note: In general, the more innocuous the substance applied to the wound the quicker it will heal. Applies even to dressings.

Source: Forest (1980).

The costs of preventing pressure sores

Prevention depends on carrying out preventing activities, either directly by health workers, or by teaching patients and their families or significant others. Allied to this is the provision of aids, although it may be suggested that in some cases buying of elaborate equipment may well be less cost-effective than employing additional health workers. Undoubtedly, the major costs of prevention lie in educating nurses and doctors, and in employing enough nurses to make the identification of those at risk, and to provide the subsequent appropriate care, a real possibility. However, if patient and family education and involvement were to become a norm in everyday nursing practice, significant increases in staff numbers may be less of a need. Thus, in economic terms, the costs of preventing the incidents of pressure sores could be minimal, apart from those that appear urgent — an increase in clinical research on preventing pressure sores.

If doctors and nurses could have more prescriptive research findings at their fingertips; would use them in their practice; and would teach patients and non-professional carers preventive strategies, much financial and human savings would be accrued.

ACTIONS TOWARDS PREVENTION

Despite the paucity of reliable advice, much can be done now to prevent pressure sores:

1. The identification of high-risk patients through the use of rating scales should become a norm of nursing practice.

2. Two-hourly position change should be the basic preventive activity.

3. Foam mattresses with polyurethane covers and firm beds should be used for high-risk patients, and should be maintained and replaced according to a planned programme.

4. Less emphasis should be placed on devices and topical applications until more evidence on their relative effectiveness is available, and more emphasis should be placed on the use of human resources.

5. Pressure-sore prevention should become a matter of concern to the whole of the multi-disciplinary clinical team, rather than purely nursing staff.

6. Patient and family education should be accepted as a legitimate nursing activity.

7. Shared care planning between nurses and patients should be a standard activity, and objectives and interventions should be written clearly and be accessible to the patient and his or her carers.

8. A more aggressive educational strategy should be pursued for both the community and health workers. For the community, pressure-sore prevention should be added to the list of health problems currently the subject of health education pamphlets, posters and other educational materials. All health workers should be made aware of the problem of pressure sores and should be educated in those aspects of prevention relevant to their role and, in particular, nurses should be taught to base their practice in this area on available knowledge, rather than on tradition.

9. Well-designed clinical research studies into the prevention of pressure sores should be encouraged and supported.

The elderly population is increasing rapidly throughout the world, and more and more people with functional limitations have many years of living ahead of them: these are the people who seem to be most susceptible to pressure sores. Although all health workers acknowledge the presence of pressure sores in the communities in which they work, and regret their occurrence, Avorn (1981) suggests that they frequently fail to contribute actively towards reversing the situation. As he asks, must we continue to contribute to the misery of these patients and their families by ignoring the problem?

REFERENCES

Agris J, Spira M 1979 Pressure ulcers: prevention and treatment. Clinical Symposia 31 (5): 1–32
Anderson K E, Jensen O, Kvorning S A, Bach e 1982 Prevention of pressure sores by identifying patients at risk. British Medical Journal 284: 1370–1371
Avorn J 1981 Nursing home infections — the context. New England Journal of Medicine 305: 759
Barbenel J C 1980 Pressure sores. Scottish Medical Journal 25: 185–186
Barbenel J C, Jordon M M, Nicol S M 1977 Incidence of pressure sores in the greater Glasgow Health Board area. Lancet 2: 548
Barbenel J C, Ferguson-Pell M W, Evans J H 1981 The chief scientist reports ... pressures produced on hospital mattresses. Health Bulletin (Edinb) 39 (1): 62–68
Bardsely C et al 1964 Pressure sores — a regimen for preventing and treating them. American Journal of Nursing 64: 82–84
Barton A A 1977 Prevention of pressure sores. Nursing Times 41: 1593–1595
Barton A, Barton M 1981 The management and prevention of pressure sores. Faber, London.
Bliss M R 1979 The use of ripple beds in hospitals. Hospital and Health Service Review 74: 190–193
Clark M O, Barbenel J C, Jordon M M, Nicol S M 1978 Nursing Times 74: 363
Cohen C 1968 Zinc sulphate and bedsores. British Medical Journal 2: 561
Cooney T C. Reuler J B 1983 Protecting the elderly patient from pressure sores. Geriatrics 38(2): 125–134
Crawford M W 1979 Pressure sores. Greater Glasgow Health Board
Daniel R K, Hall E J, MacLeod M K 1978 Pressure sores — a reappraisal. Annals of Plastic Surgery 3(1): 53–63
Daniel R K, Priest D L, Wheatley D C Etiologic factors in pressure sores: an experimental model. Arch Phys Med Rehabil 62: 492–498
Dinsdale S M 1974 Decubitus ulcers: role of pressure and friction in causation. Archives of Physical Medical Rehabilitation 55: 147–152
Dinsdale S M 1973 Decubitus ulcers in swine: light and electron microscopy study of pathogenesis. Arch Phys Med Rehabil 51: 51
Ek A C, Boman G 1982 A descriptive study of pressure sores: the prevalence of pressure sores and the characteristics of patients. Journal of Advanced Nursing 7: 51–57
Exton-Smith A N 1976 Prevention of pressure sores: monitoring mobility and assessment of clinical condition. In: Kenedi R M, Cowden J M (eds) Bedsore biomechanics. University Park Press, Baltimore.
Ferguson-Pell M W, Bell F, Evans J H 1976 In: Kenedi R M Cowden J M, Scales J T (eds) Bedsore biomechanis. Macmillan, London, p 198
Fernie G R, Dornan J 1976 The problems of clinical trial with new systems for preventing or hearling decubiti. In: Kenedi R M, Cowden J M (eds) Bedsore biomechanics. University Park Press, Baltimore.
Forrest R D 1980 The treatment of pressure sores. Journal of Internal Medical Research 8: 430–435
Galpin J E, Chow A W, Bayer A S 1976 Sepsis associated with decubitus ulcers. American Journal of Medicine 61: 364
Goldstone L A, Roberts B V 1980 A preliminary discriminant function analysis of elderly orthopaedic patients who will or will not contract a pressure sore. International Journal of Nursing Studies 17: 17–23

Goldstone L A, Goldstone J 1982 The Norton score: an early warning of pressure sores. Journal of Advanced Nursing 7: 419–426
Goswell D J 1973 An assessment tool to identify pressure sores. Nursing Research 22: 55
Judson R 1983 Pressure sores. Medical Journal of Australia 1 (9): 417–422
Kataria M S, Data A K 1982 Management of pressure areas in the elderly. Practitioner 226: 1174–1177
Kosiak M, Kubicek W G, Olsen M 1958 Evaluation of pressure as a factor in the production of ischial ulcers. Archives of Physical Medical Rehabilitation 39: 623
LaForce F M, Young L S, Bennett J V 1969 Tetanus in the United States. (1965–1966): epidemiologic and clinical features. New England Journal of Medicine 280: 569–574
Lancet 1981 Sore afflicted. (editorial) 4(2) (8236): 21–22
Ley P, Pike L A, Whitworth M A, Woodward K 1980 Effects of source, context of communication and difficulty level on the success of health educational communications concerning contraception and the menopause. Health Education Journal 1980: 47–52
Lilla J A, Friedrichs R R, Sistnes L M 1975 Flotation mattresses for preventing and treating tissue breakdown. Geriatrics 30: 71–75
Manley M T 1978 Incidence, contributory factors and costs of pressure sores. South African Medical Journal 53: 217–222
Mullholland J H, Tui C, Wright A M 1943 Protein metabolism and bed sores. Annals of Surgery 118: 1015–1023
Nightingale F 1861 Notes on Nursing — What It Is and Is Not. Appleton, New York
Norton D, Mclaren R, Exton-Smith A N 1975 An investigation of geriatric nursing problems in hospital. Churchill Livingstone. Edinburgh
Peterson N C Bittman S 1971 The epedemiology of pressure sores. Scandanavian Journal of Plastic Reconstructive Surgery 5: 62–66
Read J W 1981 Pressure ulcers in the elderly: prevention and treatment utilizing the team approach. M D State Medical Journal 30(11): 45–50
Reichel S M 1958 Shearing force as a factor in decubitus ulcers in paraplegics. Journal of the American Medical Association 166: 762–763
Reswick J B, Simoes N 1975 Application of engineering principles in management of spinal cord injured patients. Clinical Orthopedics: 112
Reuler J B: Cooney T G 1981 The pressure sore: pathophysiology and principles of management. Annasl of Internal Medicine 94: 661–666
Romm S, Tebbetts J, Lynch D, White R 1982 Pressure sores: the state of the art. Texas Medicine 78: 52–60
Rowling J T 1961 Pathological changes in mummies. Proceedings of the Royal Soceity of Medicine 54: 409–415
Shand J E, McClemont E 1979 Recent advances in the treatment of pressure sores. Paraplegia 17: 400–408
Shaw T C 1872 On so-called bed-sores in the insane. St Bartholomew's Hospital Report, London
Steffel P E S, Schenk E A, Walker S L 1980 Reducing devices for pressure sores with respect to nursing care procedures. Nursing Research 29(4): 228–230
Stewart P Wharton C W 1976 Bridging: an effective and practical method of preventive skin care of the immbolished person. South African Medical Journal 69: 1469–1473
Taylor T V, Rimmer S, Day B 1974 Ascorbic acid supplementation in the treatment of pressure sores. Lancet 1: 121–124
Tiffany C H 1977 Nursing, organisational structure and the real goals of hospitals. Unpublished Ph D Thesis, Indiana University
Walldorf S 1976 Significant changes in the care of patients with decubiti: how audit findings led to improval prevention and treatment protocols. 2: 14–23
Witowski J A: Parish L C 1982 The decubitus ulcer. International Journal of Dermatology 21(5): 259

13   J. A. Muir Gray

Education for health in old age

Once the objectives of prevention have been defined, the means by which they may be achieved can be more clearly identified. The means of prevention are numerous and varied, but they may be classified into four interrelated groups: personal preventive services, changes in the social environment, changes in the physical envirnment, and health education (see page 12). The first three of these, all of which have an educational aspect, were discussed in the first chapter; this chapter concentrates on health education.

Three types of health education may be distinguished:
1. Education about lifestyle
2. Education about the appropriate use of health and welfare services
3. Education about the ways in which decisions affecting old people are reach and ways in which they may be influenced.

Thus health education seeks not only to influence the lifestyle of elderly people; the aims of health educators are also to influence the utilisation of health services by elderly people and to accelerate the changes in the social and physical environment which are essential if old people are to be allowed to achieve their full potential.

In a survey we have recently conducted of 189 people over the age of 75 on the list of an Oxford primary care team, we were impressed by their positive beliefs and attitudes. The majority were positive about their state of health, including the majority of people over the age of 85. It is important to emphasise that their positiveness was not simply due to a failure to admit their problems because a subsequent question elicited the fact that, although 36 per cent of the subjects felt they were doing well for their age, 47 per cent made remarks that were often tinged with quiet worry, best summed up by the phrase, 'All I need is a new leg'. The positive attitude, therefore, indicates not the absence of disease but successful adaptation to disease. The majority also had positive attitudes towards growing older, but of those who said they had health problems, more than half (62 out of 112) were fatalistic about their problems and accepted them as part of the natural process of ageing. Finally, we asked the elderly people what changes they envisaged in their health in future. Of the 148 who were asked this question, 78 said they thought their health would stay the same and only 22 considered that it would get worse (Carter et al, 1984).

This survey revealed what has been demonstrated before, namely that although elderly people are often depicted as a group of ignorant, negative and pessimistic people, the majority are the opposite of this. It is thus essential that well-intentioned health educators do not convey to the public, both young and old, the image that all elderly people are like the minority whose beliefs and attitudes are negative. Some of the more common beliefs and attitudes that inhibit the old person who holds them from trying to improve his or her health are discussed in the next section of this chapter.

BELIEFS, ATTITUDES AND BEHAVIOUR

Formerly, the main aim of health education was to influence beliefs and attitudes, but in recent years there has been a shift in emphasis, and many people would now see a change in behaviour as the outcome which should be the objective of health educators. There are two principal reasons for this change in emphasis. One is that it is now appreciated that a change in beliefs and attitudes without any change in behaviour is often observed in groups exposed to health education. Thus specific measures to influence behaviour have to be included in any health education programme. For example, a programme intended to promote exercise needs not only information about the benefits of exercise and exhortations to the target group to be more active but specific advice on the frequency, duration, intensity and type of exercise, together with specific information on facilities and making these available for example by reducing charges for people who are retired. The second reason is that it is now appreciated that the apparent conflict between the behavioural approach and the approach aimed at changing beliefs and attitudes was illusory. Both approaches are needed: one effective way of influencing beliefs and attitudes is by encouraging a change in behaviour; and the most effective way of influencing behaviour is now known to be by basing health education on the beliefs and attitudes of old people.

Formerly health education was based on the assumption that people were ignorant about health and disease and required information to change their beliefs, attitudes and behaviour. This is now known to be inaccurate. Elderly people are not ignorant. They have many beliefs about health and disease, many of which have been held for decades. Admittedly some of the beliefs are not the same as those held by doctors — the beliefs which professionals call 'facts' — but the beliefs of old people are useful to them. They feel their beliefs have stood the test of time, and their confidence in them is understandable because their own survival is, to them, testimony to their correctness. Attempts to influence behaviour, therefore, have to take into account the beliefs and attitudes of elderly people.

The beliefs and attitudes of elderly people are shaped early in life but they continue to evolve in the light of daily experience, no matter how old a person may be. Three aspects of the social life continue to influence the beliefs and attitudes of older people.

The sense of immediacy

Elderly people, by and large, do not indulge in long-term planning and many, particularly those who have disabilities, live from day to day, taking each day as it comes. Many health education messages promise benefits in the future and such messages are less influential to those who view life with a foreshortened time perspective.

The sense of impotence

As people become more disabled they become more dependent, and this can result in a sense of impotence, in the feeling that all the important decisions of one's life are determined by other people. This feeling that there has been a loss of control has an influence on the individual's belief that he can determine what will happen to him, thus reducing his susceptibility to health education messages.

The sense of worthlessness

If people lose their sense of self-esteem, they are unlikely to care for themselves or their bodies as well as they did when they felt they were valuable members of society, and the sense of worthlessness and uselessness that many elders experience renders them less willing to respons to health education than they were formerly.

Thus the social and economic situation of elderly people in modern society reinforces the pessimistic and negative beliefs and attitudes that evolved in childhood and early adult life.

Common beliefs

These vary from country to country, they vary within the one country, they are different in different social classes, and they vary from one age group to another, as well as varying very much from one individual to another, but it is possible to make some generalisations because some beliefs and attitudes are commonly encountered.

'It's just my age, I suppose'

Many old people believe that everything that happens in old age is caused by the ageing process — and the consequences of this belief are serious, because the elderly person who holds such beliefs sees no reason to seek help for breathlessness or dizziness or incontinence, or for any other symptom of disease. In prevention also this belief is of fundamental importance, for if an old person believes that all the problems of old age are caused by ageing, she is unlikely to change her lifestyle or adopt any preventive measure suggested by the health educator.

Practical implications Increased emphasis has to be given to the fact that many of the problems of old age are caused not only by the ageing process but also by three other interrelated processes — loss of fitness, disease and social pressures — and so there is great scope for prevention in old age. This information should be given to old people, both as individuals and in groups, but it should not simply be broadcast at them. The first step should always be to allow the old person to express her views by asking, 'What do you think is the cause of your problem?'

It is equally important to try to change this belief in younger age groups also, particularly those young people who are training to become health workers.

'It's God's will'

In many societies old people are more influenced by religious beliefs than younger people, and in many religious disease and suffering are seen as manifestations of the will of the deity which is the focus of that religion. The religious meaning of disease varies from one religion to another but common to many religions is the idea of divine intervention: that 'God' either causes diseases to occur, or allows them to develop in some individuals and also determines who is to be spared.

The consequences of such religious beliefs vary depending upon the particular religion, but fatalism is common — a fatalistic acceptance of disease and a reluctance to believe that preventive measures suggested by a nurse, doctor or health educator can be effective in the prevention of disease.

Practical implications A sensitive approach is essential if an old person is to be encouraged to talk about this type of belief, and the main educational effort should therefore be directed towards health workers in training rather than at elderly people. Drawn from a generation that is, in many cultures, less religious than the generation that is now old, most young health workers receive a training that is based on sociology, psychology and biology and too few courses provide and adequate consideration of metaphysical or religious issues. Students in basic training should be encouraged to think about the question, 'Why should I suffer? I've led a good life, why me?' to enable the young health workers to deal sensitively with this question and its related beliefs when they meet it in practice.

For health workers and health educators who are in practice close links with local religious leaders are of great importance in keeping them sensitive to the religious dimension and aware of the metaphysical aspects of old age.

'I don't want to wear out my body'

It is now accepted that the loss of functional ability that occurs from the twenties onwards in most people is due not only to ageing but also to a loss of fitness, and fitness is at least as important to people in their seventies as it is to people in their twenties, but some older people believe that exercise is harmful and that it will accelerate the rate of degeneration. Some also believe that exercise is always contra-indicated if disease in present and that rest is therapeutic, reflecting the beliefs that formerly prevailed in medicine. The consequence of the belief that exercise is harmful is that the person who holds it will be reluctant to participate in that aspect of self care which can do most to slow the rate of physical decline — physical exercise.

Practical implications. Emphasis must be given to the benefits of physical exercise when giving old people advice on self-care and prevention. Elderly people suffering from chronic disabling diseases also need this information and because of their fears about the adverse effects of exercise need that information given in detail, not simply as the vague exhortation to 'take more exercise'.

Relatives and professional helpers also need this information (see page 91). Often a disabled old person is prevented from taking exercise because others rush in to 'help', namely taking over tasks she could do herself, thus increasing the rate of decline.

'There's no point in trying'

Some old people are very pessimistic and respond to suggestions that problems can be prevented by saying that 'it is a waste of time', or 'you should help someone who is younger, I'm too old'. In some people this reflects the belief, already discussed, that all problems are due to the ageing process. Other old people, however, hold this view although they know that the problem is theoretically preventable or treatable, because they have experienced so many disappointments and defeats that they have become hopeless and helpless.

The consequences of this belief are that the old person who holds it is unwilling to try any prevention measure.

Practical implications. The reluctance of some elderly people to try to improve their functional ability and quality of life has to be appreciated by those who are trying to help them, again emphasising the need for careful training of health workers and health educators. The old person who is apparently unwilling to try to help herself should not be dismissed as being 'awkward' or 'poorly motivated'. Possible reason for this reluctance should be considered, and the right of an old person to refuse to participate in a preventive programme should be respected. Old people, like all others, have a right to be at risk and a right to refuse offeres of help.

It is very difficult to give clear guideliness about the amount of pressure which may be exerted on an elderly person, but in general it can be said that we err too much on the side of caution and nihilism and that we should respect elderly people's ability to change and grow to a greater degree, and we should challenge their beliefs and attitudes more firmly than we do at present.

Common attitudes

Two types of attitude are particularly relevant to prevention and self-care — attitudes towards illness, of which fear is the most important, and attitudes towards health services.

Fears that are commonly encountered in speaking with elderly people may be summarised in tabular form (Table 13.1).

Obviously, elderly people may have other fears which affect their health and wellbeing, fears about poverty or debt, for example, but the fears that they have about illness and disability are of particular relevance for prevention and self-care.

In addition, many older people have different attitudes towards health and social services than younger people have, the principal reason being that in many countries elderly people grew up in an era in which these services were less easily accessible for poor people than they are today. Futhermore, in many countries access to services was controlled by a set of rules more stringent than those which apply today, and the rules were imposed by less sympathetic officials. Many elderly people thus have much lower expectations than younger people have. In addition, not all elderly people regard the services for which they are eligible as their right. Many still regard them as a favour or 'charity', and elderly people with such attitudes will be more reluctant to use services, will be more modest in their demands and more willing to accept a refusal or impoliteness or deficiencies in the service than younger people who are, in general, more assertive.

It is very difficult to change such attitudes, but it is important to try by encouraging elderly people to think about, and discuss, broader social and political issues than those which realte more obviously to their own health, such as their diet or their exercise habits. This may seem to be a shift from education about health to education about politics, but health problems in old age, like health problems at any age, have a political dimension and it is necessary to include this dimension if a programme of promoting prevention and self-care is to be comprehensive.

PROFESSIONAL BELIEFS AND ATTITUDES

The problem is not just that old people and the public have inappropriate beliefs and attitudes; many professionals also hold beliefs that are inaccurate in the light of modern research, and have attitudes that are unduly pessimistic and negative. This was clearly demonstrated in a study of attitudes to

Table 13.1 Common fears of elderly people

Fear	Nature	Consequence	Practical implications for prevention
Fear of dying	Old people are not necessarily afraid of death, but many are afraid of dying alone or in pain or of what will happen to those they themselves care for.	Anxiety.	Death and dying should be included in both professional and public education programmes.
Fear of isolation	Some immobile older people fear that, if they become independent, they will become more isolated because home care services will stop visiting. In institutions there is a fear that staff will spend less time with them.	Reluctance to participate in self-care. Dependence on others.	The prevention of isolation must be a component of prevention and self-care programmes: this can be done by increasing the number of voluntary home visits and the number of visits outside the home.
Fear of institutionalisation	Many old people are very frightened that they will be 'put in a home'.	Reluctance to discuss problems, accept offers of help.	Old people should be told that the objective of self-care and prevention is to keep them in their own homes.
Fear of dementia	Some old people assume that any memory slip is a sign of dementia.	Depression.	Education about the nature of dementia with emphasis on the fact that not every old person will develop dementia.
Fear of failure	Some elderly people have experienced so many failures as their functional ability has declined that they are reluctant to improve their lot to preclude the possibility of disappointment.	Reluctance to try preventive or self-care measures.	Some elderly people need a great deal of emotional support, in addition to information if they are to be enabled to participate in prevention or self-care.

exercise conducted in England by Jean McHeath. She found that 82 per cent of her sample of elderly people believed that exercise was 'what is wanted and needed' by old people and that it was 'important, necessary and good', whereas only 62 per cent of the professional staff had these positive attitudes. Secondly, she found that the proportion of elderly people who believed that professional staff should talk to old people about the benefits of exercise was higher than the proportion found among those staff (Table 13.2).

Of particular concern is the fact that 14 per cent of rehabilitative staff felt that talking to old people about exercise was a waste of time or unimportant.

These findings pose a serious challenge to those responsible for professional education, as the problem is not simply one of ignorance but of prejudice. Not only is professional training failing to teach professionals the facts about health in old age, it is failing to change, and sometimes reinforcing, the popular prejudices about old age.

PRIORITIES FOR HEALTH EDUCATION

Health education has to be tailored to meet the needs of the individual or community for which it is intended, but most health programmes are based on three types of topics — the transitions in life through which many elderly

Table 13.2 Percentage attitudes regarding talking to others about exercise by group (McHeath, 1983)

	Staff %	Elderly* %
Not done enough	15	52
Good to do it	8	4
Interesting/enlightening	5	1
Should do more	4	14
Important	7	14
Necessary/needed/vital	6	21
Helpful	0	4
Done if need treatment	2	1
Needs doing well	0	1
For staff to do	0	1
Don't know what should do	2	14
Only for those who know	4	1
Part of job	2	0
Pointless/daft	5	1
Not for me/not on	6	0
Not worthwhile/not good idea	5	2
Awful/useless	4	0
Unimportant/waste of time	14	1
Hard work	1	0
Feel tired	1	0
Not my job	2	0

*Includes more than one response in some cases

people pass, the risk factors in their lives and the problems that are commonly encountered.

Transitions

Individuals are always at risk at times of transition. When an individual of any age moves from one phase to another, he or she is under strain during that time of transition and this may lead to either psychological or physical problems during the time of transition or to a failure to adapt successfully to the new phase of life, or both. Most people cope successfully with transitions, but coping can be facilitated by appropriate education, both before the transition, when the transition can be foreseen, and during it. Common transitions are:

1. Bereavement, due to the effect of the death of a spouse or a friend or a pet. If death is sudden, it is obviously impossible to help the individual prepare but, where there is a protracted terminal illness, much can be done to help the person who will have to adapt.

2. Retirement, either voluntary or mandatory at a specific retirement age or precipitated through redundancy. The latter is probably the most stressful, but by its very nature offers the least opportunity for pre-retirement education.

3. The onset of disability, leading to increased isolation and dependence; this is difficult to anticipate and therefore the main educational opportunity arises during the early phase of the disabling illness.

Education can help people maintain their health through these transitions and adapt successfully to the new phase.

Risk factors

The risk factors that predispose to disease in old age are not clearly understood, largely because the natural history of old age is not clearly understood. Nevertheless it is possible to identify a number of risk factors that can be influenced by an educational approach:

1. Physical inactivity.

2. Mental inactivity, though less closely studied than physical activity, is also harmful.

3. Inadequate dietary intake.

4. The receipt of long-term medication is a risk factor, but one that should be primarily the focus of professional education; too often the elderly person is blamed for failing to comply with medical advice when the fault is primarily that of the professionals.

5. Cigarette smoking remains a risk factor in old age, and elderly smokers should be advised to stop, to prevent further decline in lung function, to improve their symptoms and to prepare them to cope more effectively with

acute respiratory infections.

These are some of the risk factors that can be influenced by education.

Problems

Health education is conventionally defind as being associated with the primary prevention of disease, but education also has an important part to play when a problem has developed, and this type of education, sometimes called patient education, should be incorporated in any programme of education for health in old age. Everyone who develops a problem needs education, but some problems require more information than others, for example:

1. Having had a stroke
2. Caring for a disabled relative, particularly a relative or spouse with dementia
3. Having diabetes
4. Having a problem with sleeping, either insufficient sleep or anciety about sleeping
5. Being depressed
6. Having a leg ulcer
7. Having arthritis
8. Being blind
9. Being deaf
10. Having stress incontinence.

In some cases education will be an alternative to drug treatment, for example in the management of depression or sleeping problems, in others education complements and supplements the therapeutic intervention.

THE MEANS OF HEALTH EDUCATION

Little is known about the most effective means of health education in old age. The mass media have a part to play in changing beliefs and attitudes, for example by repeating the simple message that 'it's never too late'. However, the most effective intervention is probably personal, the education of one person by another. The scope for education during the contacts elderly people make with health and social services is now appreciated and the potential of the consultation is being more effectively exploited as professionals recognise that the consultation should be used not only to solve the presenting problem but also as an opportunity for exploring other issues, including the promotion of health.

It is also being appreciated that the education approach to elderly people, whether in a consultation or in a formal educational setting such as pre-retirement education, requires a different approach from the pedagogic approach derived from the schoolroom. As Allin Coleman demonstrated in the Health Education Council's pre-retirement programme, adults do wish

224 PREVENTION OF DISEASE IN THE ELDERLY

information about their body, health and disease but education also has to be based on the unique experience of each individual and to be associated not simply with the acquisition of skills and information but with the personal development of that individual. The field of adult education is expanding quickly and there is information based on well-tested theories to allow the development of effective educational programmes.

The problem is not primarily a lack of information; it is the unwillingness of professionals to use the information that is available. Too often elderly people are approached with inaccurate material in an inappropriate style. Fortunately, the ineffectiveness of the approach means that much of the inaccurate information does not influence the old people exposed to it, but this is cold comfort. There is information that is important for old people, and there are techniques for imparting it effectively and enjoyably. The challenge is to encourage professionals to adopt these techniques.

A STRATEGY FOR HEALTH EDUCATION

It is obviously appropriate to aim health education at elderly people themselves, but it is essential to recognise that elderly people are not a homogeneous group and that anyone who is planning a health education

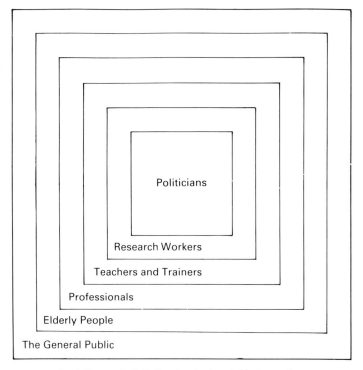

Fig. 13.1 Groups that influence the beliefs and attitudes of elderly people

programme for a population of old people has to be prepared to develop a number of different programmes for different groups of elderly people, for example for active elderly people, for the housebound and for those who live in institutions. It is, however, equally important to develop health education not only for elderly people themselves but for all the other groups of people who influence the beliefs and attitudes of older people. These groups may be represented diagrammatically (Fig. 13.1).

It is necessary not only to develop educational programmes for each group but also to develop an integrated strategy which links these individual programmes. Two principles of integration which are of particular importance are:

1. Each group needs to be informed what the group that is immediately central to it is doing; for example, elderly people need to be informed not only that exercise is beneficial but that the professionals in training are now also being taught this.

2. Each group needs to be aware of the education being offered to all the groups peripheral to it; for example, research workers need to be informed about the education being directed at the general public, at elderly people, at professionals and at teachers and trainers, in the hope that this will influence their research priorities.

Elderly people do not exist in isolation. They exist in society, being influenced by, and influencing, other groups. They cannot, and should not, be expected to change in isolation, and education for health in old age should not simply be directed at people who are growing old or who are old; everybody, including highly-trained professionals, require education to help them cope with the major challenge that is posed by the ageing of our population.

REFERENCES

Carter A, Garland J, NcLennan N, Thoroughgood M, Gray J A M 1984 Drug use and health in old age. Oxfordshire Health Authority

McHeath J A 1983 Activity, health and fitness in old age. Croom Helm, London

Index

Ageing, 4–11
 balance, 78–81, 118–122
 body composition, 178–180
 bone, 96–97
 energy intake, 182–183
 neurophysiological changes, 161
Alcohol abuse
 nutritional problems, 187
 osteoporosis, 109
 postural hypotension, 123
 stroke, 148
Alzheimer's disease, 16
Anaemia, 185, 187
Anxiety, 88
Aspirin, 142
Assessment, 27–28
Attitudes towards old people, 19–20, 28–30, 62, 92–93, 219–221

Behaviour modification, 32–33
Behavioural problems, 28–34
Bereavement, 61, 164, 166–167
 and suicide, 173

Calcium deficiency, 104–105, 184
Cancer, 181
Case finding, 11, 51–63
Chiropody, 13
Cigarette smoking, 6, 101, 104, 146
Cohort studies, 7–9
Cognitive training, 30–31, 51–63
 depression, 168
Compliance, *see* Iatrogenic disease
Confusion caused by drugs, 68
Cost effectiveness, 2
 osteoporosis, 99
 pressure sores, 209–211
 screening, 60–62
 stroke, 150
Cross sequential analysis, 9
Cycling, 83

Dependency, prevention of, 18–37
Depression, 156–177

Diabetes mellitus, 146
Diet, *see* Nutritional problems
Disability, 21–25, 82
 depression, 162–163
 nutritional problems, 187
 stroke, 135–137
District nurse, 74
Drugs, *see* Iatrogenic disease

Effects of prevention, 2–4, 9–11, 16, 57
Environmental health officer, 127
Environmental measures, 14, 34–35
Ethical aspects of prevention, 14–16, 91–93
Exercise, 78–94
 falls, 127
 osteoporosis, 105–106
 pressure sores 202
 stroke, 148

Falls, 114–129
Family breakdown, 28–30, 38–50
Family medicine, *see* General practice
Fractures, 95–99

General practice, 13, 60–62, 64–66, 74–75

Health beliefs, 15–16, 57, 214–219
 exercise, 79–82
Health education, 12, 89, 214–225
Health visitor, 60–62, 74–75
High blood pressure, 137–142
Home helps, 76
Housing problems, 14, 45, 48
 falls, 118, 127
Hyperlipidaemia, 147

Iatrogenic disease, 64–77, 143, 170
 confusion, 68
 diuretics, 69
 osteoporosis, 109
 postural hypotension, 123, 140
Inactivity, *see* Exercise
Incontinence, 196, 202
Intellectual impairment, 5, 7, 21, 30–32, 74

Isolation, 61, 165
   depression, 165
   nutritional problems, 187
   suicide, 173

Longitudinal studies, 6–9
Meals on wheels, 187–188

Nuffield Provincial Hospitals Trust, 53
Nutritional problems, 178–193
   ascorbic acid deficiency, 183, 186, 187, 209
   calcium deficiency, 104–105, 184
   hyperlipidaemia, 147
   osteomalacia, 109–110, 184
   osteoporosis, 101, 104–105
   pressure sores, 207
   protein deficiency, 185
   vitamin deficiencies, 109–110, 184, 186–187

Obesity, 110, 146
Occupational therapy, 13
Oestrogens, 106–109
Osteomalacia, 109–110, 184
Osteoporosis, 10, 95–113, 184

Parkinson's disease, 16
Patient education, 223
Pharmacist, 75
Physiotherapy, 13
Postural hypotension, 122–125
Poverty, 13, 19, 48, 61
   depression, 164
   nutritional problems, 187
   stroke, 147
Pressure sores, 194–213
Priestley, JB, 90
Primary prevention, 11
Professional education, 219

Protein deficiency, 185, 207, 209
Psychotropic drugs, 68

Reality orientation, 30–32
Residential care, 62
Risk factors, 60–62, 222–223

Salt intake, 140
Samaritans, 174
Screening, 11, 51–63
Secondary prevention, 11, 51–63
   depression, 167
   pressure sores, 207
Self care, 67
Skill, 87
Social workers, 75
Stamina, 85
Strength, 86
Stroke, 130–155
   anticoagulants, 144
   atrial fibrillation, 145
   diabetes, 146
   obesity, 146
   polycythaemia, 146
   smoking, 146
Suicide, 156–177
Suppleness, 86

Tertiary prevention, 12
Transient ischaemic attack, 130–155
Tuberculosis, 10

Unfitness, *see* Exercise

Vascular disease, 187
Vitamin deficiency, 109–111, 184, 186–187
Vitamin D deficiency, 109–110, 184, 186